Hospital Gowns
and
Other Embarrassments

L GOWNS

AND

OTHER

EMBARRASSMENTS

A TEEN GIRL'S GUIDE TO HOSPITALS

Michael W. Perry

INKLING BOOKS   SEATTLE   2012

Description

With needles, strangers, and embarrassing situations, hospitals can be scary places, particularly if you're a teen girl. I can't do anything about those needles. That's up to your doctor. But I can tell you how to change those strangers into friends and how to avoid that embarrassment with great skill. That's because I cared for girls just like you at one of the nation's top children's hospitals. This book tells you how to make your hospital stay much more enjoyable.

Copyright Notice

Dedication

Dedicated to teen girls everywhere.

Library Cataloging Data

Title: *Hospital Gowns and Other Embarrassments: A Teen Girl's Guide to Hospitals*
Author: Michael W. Perry (1948–).
Description: 146 pages.
Size: 6 x 9 x 0.34 inches, 229 x 152 x 9 mm. Weight: 0.5 pounds, 225 grams.
Library of Congress Control Number: 2012921981 (paper edition).
BISAC Subject Headings:
REF015000—REFERENCE / PERSONAL & PRACTICAL GUIDES
HEA024000—HEALTH & FITNESS / WOMEN'S HEALTH
MED058080—MEDICAL / NURSING / PEDIATRIC & NEONATAL
ISBN for paperback: 978-1-58742-066-5
ISBN for ePub: 978-1-58742-067-2 (iBookstore)
ISBN for Kindle: 978-1-58742-068-9 (Amazon)
ISBN for Smashwords: 978-1-58742-069-6 (Others)

Publisher Information

Print edition published in the United States of America on acid-free paper.
First edition. Second printing
Publisher: Inkling Books, Seattle, December, 2012.
Internet: http://www.InklingBooks.com/

CONTENTS

1. This Book Is For You

If you're a teenaged girl who's about to enter a hospital—or perhaps already there—then this book was written especially for you. And no, it's not one of those scary 'What to know before your surgery' pamphlets that a hospital might give you. It's true that I'll be mentioning things such as IVs, sutures and even spinal taps, but they're just incidentals. This book is about something that rarely gets mentioned in those pamphlets or by most doctors and nurses. It's almost a secret they wish no one would talk about. Well, I will be talking about it and offering clear and practical advice, so when you enter that hospital, you'll be prepared for what you find there and know what to do.

Unfortunately, it's not easy to come up with a word that describes what I'll be discussing. Some might call it privacy, but for others that seems cold, like something a lawyer might say. Modesty also fits, but that has an old fashioned ring. It brings to mind "Little House on the Prairie" reruns with girls in ankle-length dresses running down flower-covered hillsides. You know quite well that you won't be wearing ankle-length dresses in a hospital. Instead, it'll be a gown that covers embarrassing little, hence the book's title *Hospital Gowns and Other Embarrassments*. That's why I'll favor the word embarrassment. We all know what that means. It's when something happens that we'd rather not have happened, something we later remember with regret. That happens all too often in a hospital, particularly if you're a teen-aged girl.

Little Min's Story

Perhaps the best illustration comes from a young girl that I took care of for several days. I'll call her Min, a name the Chinese give to daughters who are especially sensitive and quick with their feelings, because that's precisely what Min was like.

Min was Asian and tiny even for a girl of eleven. I've forgotten the details, but she had something wrong with her back so serious that she not only required a major surgery, afterward she had to spend most of every day in a body cast that went from her neck to just above her knees. In that cast, the only parts of her she could move were her head, her arms and her lower legs. Scary isn't it? It's almost as bad as being tied up.

People in her situation get sores if they are left in one position too long, so it was my job to go to her bed every two hours and flip her over. If she was face down, I turned her face up and vice versa. Remember, when she's in that near-full-body cast, she can do nothing to stop me. She must have felt very helpless.

That was why, when I came up to her bed, a frightened little Min looked up at me with pure terror filling her young, pretty eyes. Now, except for my beard, I'm a rather ordinary looking guy, so I'm not used to scaring anyone. But I knew why she was afraid.

For practical reasons, her body cast had two openings, one on each side. I knew that because, for about an hour each day, she was out of the cast to allow it to dry out. When I came up to her, she was afraid of something that happens many times a day in almost any hospital. A member of the staff, needing to do something to a patient, finds a sheet in the way, and simply sweeps it aside, even though it's the only covering that patient has. I suspect some of our staff were treating Min that way. To be fair, they had a lot to do and didn't have much time. I'll talk more about that later. Just keep in mind that when that sheet was swept aside, Min felt most embarrassed.

Making matters still worse, she happened to be in the most exposed-to-the-outside bed in the entire hospital. It was next to a large, second-floor picture window just above the hospital's main entrance. Even though a curtain was drawn around her bed, that curtain could be swept aside in a second. So Mia had good reason to be afraid, even if the person caring for her was a woman.

Now, if I'd been caring for a boy I knew well enough to know he didn't care, I'd sweep that sheet aside too. I had as much reason to be in a hurry as anyone else. But she was a girl and with girls I never did that. With any girl, I would be careful. With Min, seeing how she felt, I was extra careful, flipping her slowly and stopping every few seconds to adjust that sheet so nothing showed.

Unfortunately, despite all the times I flipped her, Min never understood what I was doing. For all she knew, this time might be the one where I might rush up, rip off her sheet, reveal one of those openings, and then casually flip her over, revealing the other. Trapped in that cast, there would be nothing she could do. That was why she was afraid of me, and that's where I failed her. I should have bent down close, looked into her eyes, and whispered, "Don't worry. I've done this lots of times. I'll be careful. Nothing will show."

Yes, my silence does have an excuse of sorts. Although at the time I'd worked at that top-ranked children's hospital for over a year and a half, taking care of some of its sickest patients, nothing in my training had taught me how to calm her fears. I knew how to talk about pain and the fear of pain. I knew how to deal with the nausea that our chemotherapy caused. I could even deal with the intensely emotional issues that surround dying. I had taken care of dying children, and in some cases, I was the only one on staff providing their final care. But strange as it sounds, I was never taught how to deal with embarrassment or how to prevent it—nothing at all. What I learned, I learned in a most fumbling fashion on my own, so much so that I'm almost embarrassed to recount the tale here. But for your sake, I will.

Even worse, there was unfortunately little in the culture of my hospital—or I suspect most modern hospitals—to encourage me to deal kindly with Min's fears of embarrassment. Among some hospital staff, those feelings were usually ignored and only taken seriously when a patient raised them—something that Min was far too shy and frightened to do. Later, I'll explain why that's so.

Yes, it is true that, in the great depth of her fears, Min was exceptional. Few of the other girls I saw in my hospital were quite as afraid of exposure as she was. But many do have feelings like hers. So, if you find yourself sympathizing with little, encased-in-plaster Min, then this book is for you. In it, I'll tell you why hospitals treat patients the way they do and offer some practical advice about how to take control of your situation and avoid most, if not all, embarrassments. You can learn to live with that embarrassing hospital gown and all that goes with

About this Book

Now for a few words about this book. First, everyone you'll read about here was an actual patient of mine, and all the events happened exactly as described. I did take a little liberty with certain, non-critical parts of the stories. While the descriptions of these girls are the best I can recall, specific details may not be precise. A girl I describe as thirteen may have actually been fourteen, for instance, or someone I say has blonde hair may have actually had light-brown hair. The need to make these girls and their circumstances vivid, I felt, was more important than the limitations of my memory. I want you to see these girls as if you were standing beside me as I made my rounds, feeling much as they felt. I can't do that if I describe them as "from thirteen to fifteen" or "with blonde or maybe light-brown hair." Also, in keeping with medical practice, all the names here are stand-ins for their real names with the exception of Binky, a wonderful little guy whose nickname I've kept to honor his memory.

Second, although I wish it didn't have to be true, some of these stories are grim. I'm not trying to make you sad. It's simply that many of the patients that I cared for were either dying or facing the serious possibility of doing so. Although I do think girls in such situations deserve special kindness, that's not my main purpose here. Every girl in a hospital deserves the best of care. No, I'm simply describing my experiences. The children's hospital where I worked took in the most seriously ill children and teens over a four-state region, and the positions I held meant I often cared for the sickest of them. These were simply my patients.

Third, as I write this, much of what I'll be saying is a near-taboo topic within medicine (what doctors do) and nursing (what nurses do). Because I believe that problems aren't solved by saying nothing, I intend, with your help, to break that silence. Embarrassment, I believe, is as important to many patients as pain. Hospitals are careful to deal with any pain you might suffer. They should be just as careful with embarrassment. That's the broad message of this book.

Fourth—and where I need your understanding the most—some of the details that I'll describe here are, to put it frankly, embarrassing. That's the theme of this book, so there's no way I can avoid that. Talking about embarrassment can be embarrassing. I do hope that by being frank, I'll help prepare you for your hospital stay and make it a much better one. A hospital isn't a five-star hotel, so you need to be prepared. Reading about what can happen here should help prepare you.

Fifth, while this book's central topic is embarrassment and how to avoid it, much of what I suggest here applies equally well to other areas. If you're frightened by needles, for instance, this book will help you win the sympathy of hospital staff, with perhaps some gentler treatment and fewer pokes. Although this book was written for teen girls, older women or even boys and men may find much of what I say useful.

Last, keep in mind that, to cover every possibility, I tell how to deal some situations that aren't likely to happen to you. You'll probably be quite happy with the staff who care for you, men as well as women. But for that small minority of cases, I tell you what to do if you get stuck with a creepy guy or how to deal with the hospital administration if something really unpleasant happens. If you find those discussions unsettling, skip over them for now. You probably won't need them. But keep this book available just in case you do.

Next, I describe myself in more detail, along with what I did at that hospital.

Hospital Gowns and Other Embarrassments

2. INTRODUCING MYSELF

At this point, I should introduce myself. Years ago, several situations in which I was almost killed while mountain climbing motivated me to take an Emergency Medical Technician course at a community college. I wanted to be prepared for anything that might happen in the wilderness. That, in turn, led to working night shift at a children's hospital, a hospital so important that it was the primary referral center for seriously ill children for almost one-fourth the land area of the U.S. (including Alaska). In current rankings, it's one of the top ten children's hospitals in the country.

There I was assigned to the medical unit, where I worked at night as a pediatric aide alongside a nurse taking care of children from one to nine years old whose treatment was medical rather than surgical. Typically, these kids were getting medicines through IVs in their veins. Emotionally, it was a simple role to play. They were children, so the nurse and I served as substitutes for their mothers and fathers. We calmed them down, eased their fears, and cared for them like parents do.

Working on Hem-Onc

My primary assignment, however, was to a set of rooms on the medical unit that treated Hem-Onc patients. At that time, these were children from birth to nine years old who had some form of blood disorder (*Hem*atology) or cancer (*Onc*ology), typically leukemia, which is a cancer of the blood and the most common cancer among children. My position was perhaps the most difficult aide position in the hospital, and I shared it with a third-year nursing student. Between the two of us, we kept Hem-Onc staffed with an experienced aide seven nights a week. We checked their vital signs (temperature along with heart and breathing rates). We also took care of their personal needs. Sometimes, when their parents weren't there, we fed and rocked them to sleep.

Hem-Onc was grim work. The chemotherapy we used to treat leukemia left our kids looking like survivors of some horrible concentration camp. Many were so weak they could hardly stand and had pale skin with only a few wisps of hair. Things are better today, but at that time the treatment was brutal. To get rid of those evil leukemic cells, our chemotherapy pushed their blood counts to dangerously low levels. To save them, we had to almost kill them.

The outcomes were often unhappy. Despite all our efforts, on average a third of the children we cared for would die. And yet despite that, I found the work so filled with meaning, I preferred it to caring for the much healthier kids elsewhere on the medical unit. The other kids would almost certainly get well. We merely made their sickness a bit shorter and less uncomfortable. With the kids on Hem-Onc, if I did my job well, I could make the difference between life and death for some little boy or girl. You'll find their stories in a companion book I've written called *Nights with Leukemia*. This book covers issues that had originally been a part of that book, until I realized that these embarrassing experiences didn't belong there.

There was another emotionally satisfying benefit to working Hem-Onc. Because our kids were typically there for weeks if not months, I got to know them very well. There were only seven rooms, about the most a nurse and I could handle, so I was always working with the same group of kids night after night and week after week. Later on the teen unit, I would become frustrated rotating between the unit's three clusters of rooms. I'd just be getting to know one set of patients, including perhaps one with leukemia, when my two days off would come. When I returned, I'd almost always go to a different cluster with different teens. It might be a month before that rotation took me back to some of those same patients. That left me feeling out of touch with them. I liked getting to know my patients—in fact, I liked my all patients. I made a point of doing that. If you'd been my patient, I'd have liked you.

Moving to Teens

Most of this book concerns those later experiences working days on the hospital's teen unit, so I should tell you how I got there. After almost a year and a half of working nights on Hem-Onc—from February of one year to May of the next—I was exhausted. I'd worked nights with three sets of nurses, and the third set was now moving on to other shifts. Odd as it sounds, it wasn't the dying. I could accept that. I did all I could to give those children the best possible chance at life and, failing that, the best possible death. I had done what I could for them. There was no reason to feel bad about that.

No, what was exhausting me were other physical and emotional issues. Night work is brutal on the body. Even more important, senseless clashes between the nursing staff had reached the point where the care of the kids was being affected in harmful ways. After one boy almost died from a morphine overdose, I decided to leave a rapidly worsening situation I could not change.

That's when a different position opened up. Occasionally on night shift I'd floated to the teen unit, and a friend there persuaded me to apply for an open slot on day shift. I was accepted. Fortunately, one thing wouldn't change. I would still care for patients battling cancer, including leukemia. That's why *Nights with Leukemia* goes on to tell their stories. This book tells a different set of stories, mostly drawn from the half of each day that I spent working with teen girls. This is as much their story as mine, and I hope you find it helpful. To those girls I offer a much belated thanks for putting up with me and my many blunders.

But first things first. Before I describe my experiences with teen girls, I must describe two experiences I had with teen girls while I was still working Hem-Onc. They shaped my later work on the teen unit in ways I'm still trying to understand.

3. INNOCENT MARIA

This fourteen-year-old girl's admission was a great break in our routine. The medical unit on which I was working nights took care of non-surgical children between one and nine years of age, while the Hem-Onc cluster to which I was usually assigned took care of those from birth to nine with some form of cancer, usually leukemia. It wasn't pleasant work, but it had a meaning and purpose I've never found anywhere else.

The hospital called me a pediatric aide. In today's terms terms I was a nursing technician (a skilled nursing assistant) working alongside Hem-Onc's sole night nurse. The work was hard. Times beyond counting, I held and comforted a child vomiting from our chemotherapy. When that happened, I would tell myself that what we were doing wasn't evil, that it was their only hope.

I would also remind myself that working there made it easy to be good. Any difficulty in my life was nothing in comparison to the stark futures these children faced. Exhausted from missed sleep—"Stay alert, this little boy could die." Having trouble with a new nurse—"Cope with it, this little girl could die." Every time I brought out that demanding scale, the decision always fell on the side of the child. In a strange sort of way, that most terrible of situations made it easy to be good.

Liking Maria

The stress meant that it was wonderful, from time to time, to glimpse medicine's less grim side. That particular night almost every bed in the hospital was filled, so when Maria, a cute, dark-eyed, fourteen-year-old Hispanic girl arrived with acute appendicitis, the usual age limitation was waved, and she was sent to a normally empty room next to Hem-Onc that'd originally been intended for pediatric dialysis. Her condition wasn't serious enough that she was in pain, but the hospital wasn't taking chances. Her operation was scheduled for the next day.

Almost certainly facing surgery for the first time, Maria was too nervous to sleep. By good fortune, it was a slow night, so both the nurse and I talked with her and reassured her. She was gentle, quiet, and polite, an exceptionally sweet, innocent, and modest girl trying to be brave. I found myself liking her and that felt good. On Hem-Onc, liking a child always came with the bitter realization that he or she might die. This girl wasn't going to die. She was young, healthy and full of life. One quick little surgery and she'd be home well.

Nights rarely dealt with new admissions, so my nurse, who was a new graduate, was delighted that this time she got to write the nursing assessment. Later, I had a chance to read it and was impressed with but one exception. At one point, she wrote that this fourteen-year-old girl "denies recent sexual activity." I felt like marching over, pointing to that passage, and telling her, "You make her sound like an out-of-work prostitute and a dishonest one at that."

Be careful who you criticize, because that criticism can turn around and bite you. That's what happened that night. An image flashed into my mind, and I realized that I'd treated that young teen girl far worse than the nurse I was about to attack. She'd merely written a bit of medical boilerplate that the girl would never read. I'd done something much worse.

Girls and Bedpans

It happened the first time my nurse and I were in the overflow room with Maria and another girl. I was with the five-year-old, when Maria asked the nurse for a bedpan. The nurse could have taken care of her request in a few seconds. But as always happened in those cases, she said that I'd take care of it and left the room. When you're in a hospital, don't forget that. Most nurses see themselves as skilled professionals. They don't do bedpans when they can avoid them. Bedpans are for assistants like me. If we're around, we get the job—even if we're a guy and you're a girl. Hospitals can be embarrassing places.

Take care of it I did. About a minute later, when I finished with the younger girl, I walked over and slipped the bedpan in place. Then I pulled down Maria's sheets, flipped up her gown and yanked her panties below her knees. Yes, the room was fairly dark, and I covered her with the sheets in the same motion in which I pulled down her panties. I'd done that hundreds of times, so what I did was smooth and fast. The faster I worked, the sooner a little child could get back to sleep, and I could go on to other things. Even at night, hospitals are busy places.

Also, keep in mind that sort of thing lay at the center of my job. In fact, at times when I was feeling glum, I'd tell nurses that my work was 'pee-pee checks.' They'd laugh, because that was almost true. On the medical unit, a nurse spent her time pumping liquids into kids, which is why our nurses complained of taking care of IV pumps rather than kids. I spent my time dealing with those liquids when they came back out—measuring their volume and PH (for those on chemotherapy), as well as running other tests as ordered. I changed so many diapers, I joke that I should be exempt from another diaper change for the rest of my life. And for kids beyond number—boys and girls alike—I'd done something similar to what I'd done with Maria. I'd flipped up their gowns, pulled down their underpants and placed them on a bedpan or a toilet. That's why the nurse referred Maria to me. Bedpans were what I did.

But the more I thought about what I'd done, the more uncomfortable I became. Yes, I worked in a hospital where staff, male and female, did what I'd done times beyond counting for patients of both sexes and all ages. That was normal, and with kids of the age we were caring for on the medical unit, it wasn't really an issue. But Maria wasn't a four-year-old. She was a sexually mature, fourteen-year-old girl, and I was a guy she'd never seen before that evening. There was no getting around the fact that I should not have treated her that callously. I was the one who'd treated her like a prostitute.

Two Different Worlds

To understand the wrongness as I saw it that night, realize that, as that evening began, Maria and I lived in two distinctly different worlds. She lived in the broad outside world. I lived in a narrow and specialized subset of that world called a modern children's hospital. Despite her physical presence in our hospital, emotionally and psychologically she remained in a world where guys didn't do things like that—or got arrested if they tried. However she might accept my behavior on one level—"This is what happens in hospitals"—at another level it was a violation of who she was as a young woman. Nor did I regard what I did as OK simply because another woman—my nurse that night—regarded it as OK. She was as much a part of specialized world as I. We shared the same blindness.

No, I'm not saying that deeds like those are wrong in themselves. Sick people need to have their needs taken care of in a hospital, including bedpans. There are practical reasons why both men and women need to be involved in that care. I'm not arguing that above some age women should be handling all the more private needs of female patients and men those of male patients. I know that would be utterly unworkable. I'd simply concluded that what I did needed to change in some way.

Older Girls

Change I did. After Maria, I adjusted how I handled older girls—those from seven and up. Why seven? Because I'd noticed that at about that age my Hem-Onc boys and girls developed a modesty that made my work easier. Boys started keeping a urinal in the bed with them. Girls began to ask their mother for a bedpan. On my rounds I'd find a filled urinal or bedpan waiting for those 'pee pee checks.' So for those older girls I took the time to treat them differently. It wasn't perfect, but it was better. In fact, it resembled the hospital's own policy of not having boys and girls from ten and up in the same multi-bed room. I'll explain the reason for that later.

Although I didn't realize it at the time. That night was a watershed. Before that night, I'd been an aide who merely happened to be a guy. After that night, I became a guy who was also an aide. If my guyness mattered to those I was caring for—and it certainly did—then it needed to matter to me.

4. Gentle Christy

Thanks to sweet and innocent Maria, I'd begun to see myself, not just as a member of the hospital's medical staff, but as someone whose 'guyness' was an unalterable factor in the care I gave. More and more, I began to see myself not just as a caregiver but as a caregiver who was also a guy.

Soon, another girl just a little older would profoundly shape my thinking, although her circumstances could not have been more different. It began at report time, when the evening nurse would describe the patients my nurse and I would be taking care of that night. As soon as she began to tell us about Christy's plight, I resolved to do everything I could to ease her death. If it needed to be done, I would do it. At that moment, I didn't realize all that meant.

Christy's Plight

Christy had a inoperable brain tumor, so medically, there was nothing we could do for her. Just shy of fifteen, she was outside our normal age range, but her transfer to Hem-Onc wasn't surprising. We knew how to handle dying, so from time to time we received patients who came to us simply to die. But in Christy's case, there was an infinitely sadder reason.

Christy came to us because every single nurse on the teen unit refused to care for her anymore. And no, they weren't objecting to Christy herself. I've never had a quieter, gentler, more easy to care for patient in my entire life. Despite all she was going through, I never heard a word of complaint from her. She was absolutely wonderful.

The problem lay with her mother. In their grief, some people become angry. Christy's mother was not only extremely angry, she was venting her anger at the most ready target—her daughter's nurses. She seemed to have a peculiar talent for getting under people's skin. The nurses on the teen unit could no longer endure the mother. She'd wrecked her relationship with every one of them, so Hem-Onc was Christy's last hope. We were the only other place in the hospital accustomed to caring for people in her situation. I felt like my heart had been ripped out. No one who is dying should have to go through that.

At report, I also learned something else. It was clear that she needed no nursing care, and I knew that meant—I would take on all her care. The nurses on Hem-Onc were marvelous at caring for dying children. But for reasons I could never quite understood, they shied away from a dying child who required no nursing expertise. Order a simple IV drip, and they'd be in and out of the room through the night. Give them a child that needed only the care that was among my job skills, and they remained away, leaving everything to me. On one occasion, I doubt my nurse even visited a dying little boy's room until I told her that he had died. Perhaps it was their image of themselves as healers that required that they be doing something medical. Without that, they were lost. And I was right—that's precisely what happened with Christy.

Caring for Christy

After report, I went to Christy. I told her I'd be taking care of her and that, if she needed anything, she need only press the call button, and I would come as fast as possible. I also told her that if there was anything she'd rather I not do, to just tell me and I would get the nurse. Unfortunately, as I mentioned above, it was a nurse she'd rarely see. To myself, I also resolved that, no matter how busy I was elsewhere, I would never give any indication of that to her. I could do nothing to alter the madness that afflicted her mother. But her mother wasn't staying overnight—a wonderful blessing. In those few hours I could surround her with as much kindness and peace as I could. She deserved that.

Christy came on a Thursday. I remember that because the evening nurse told us that the following Thursday was her fifteenth birthday. I'm sure I was not the only one who thought, "that's when she'll die." But the fact that it was a Thursday also meant something that'd help me sort out my thoughts. At that time, I had an arrangement with the nursing student who shared my position. I worked weekdays, and she worked Friday and Saturday evenings, which fit better with her class schedule. She'd be taking care of Christy the next two nights, and I'd return for the following week. That gave me time to think.

I needed time, because one part of the care I would provide was bothering me immensely, "She's a teen-aged girl," I told myself. "I'm a guy in his thirties that she's never seen before. Her tumor has left her almost helpless, able to use her arms and to twist from side to side but not much else. I'll have to do everything else for her." How would she feel being handled by a guy she hardly knew? Her terrible cancer, her berserk mother, the expulsion from the teen unit, and now me. Was I to be the final indignity in her life? The thought made me sick.

Over the weekend, I remembered my brush with hospital care a couple of years before when I'd been in a car accident and medics had rushed me to the city's primary trauma center. With only cuts and strained muscles, I was discharged a few hours later, attended by no one but a bored intern. But I still remembered the rush of attention I received when I first arrived, with staff starting an IV and placing pads for an EKG monitor simultaneously. They also stripped off my clothes, replacing them with a gown, and I recall appreciating a nurse who glanced away in the brief moment between my clothes and my gown.

Hospital Gowns and Other Embarrassments

I promised myself that I'd do something similarly kind for Christy. If I'd noticed that glance in the middle of a life-threatening emergency, I knew that Christy, a teen-aged girl, helpless and alone in the middle of the night, would be watching me carefully, tuned in to every glance of my eyes, every move I made, and even the tone of my voice. If she decided she could trust me, all would be well. But I had to be worthy of her trust. Fortunately, that worked. She trusted me, and we became friends.

One by one, the nights passed. When I would come around, Christy was quiet, and I didn't intrude. It was hard to know what to talk about, so I said little. We couldn't talk about her future, because she had none. We couldn't talk about her past, because I didn't know where the painful memories might lie. We certainly couldn't talk about her family.

Looking back, I wished I'd slipped in a question about what flower she liked best. With only a little effort, I could have gotten everyone on the medical and teen units to sign a card. No one had any ill will toward her. Then I could have attached that card to a bundle of her favorite flowers as a gift from everyone at the hospital. A gift like that was something she desperately needed. The rooms of most dying kids—and especially teen girls—are filled with flowers, balloons, and stuffed animals. Hers was as bare and empty as a tomb, the result of her mother's scorched-earth behavior. Sadly, the thought never came to me.

I never saw Christy sleep. What she seemed to want most was time to dwell in her own thoughts. Only at night did she have peace. If she stayed awake then, she could sleep during what must have been a hellish day when her mother was yelling at our nurses. And yell that mother did. Within a few days, almost every nurse working Hem-Onc during days and evenings had come to hate the mother. She had a talent for making enemies. The only exception was night shift, which was spared her presence. In the end, that would prove a great blessing.

Breathe Christy, Breathe

Every night as I watched, Christy seemed to grow more quiet and withdrawn. Finally, Wednesday evening came, the eve of her fifteenth birthday. When my nurse and I arrived, the evening nurse told us she was in a coma. A few minutes after midnight, I went into her room. "She's fifteen now," I said to myself.

Turning from side to side is important with unconscious patients. She was on her right side, so I turned her on her left. She stopped breathing. Troubled as her family relations where, I told myself, they still had a right to be here when she died. I shook her shoulders gently and whispered, "Breathe Christy, breathe." She began to breath again. That would be my last act of kindness. I'd given her a few more hours of life.

Her mother arrived about half an hour later. That's when I had reason to be thankful. Christy's nights had been filled with kindness and peace, just as I had hoped. Almost alone among the nursing staff, Christy's nurse and I had not met the mother and thus weren't angry at her. There was something else that mattered too. The nurse I was working with that night might not have been the most technically skilled, but she was marvelous with people. About four a.m., Christy stopped breathing again, and the mother began to scream for us to "Do something." Instead, that wonderful nurse gently held the mother and kept repeating, "Let her go. Let her go."

I'd been afraid that, because of me, Christy's last days would be marred. That hadn't happened. She died being cared for a friend who simply happened to be a guy. And I knew that recognizing I was a guy and making the proper adjustments had made all the difference. For that I could thank sweet little Maria. With Maria, I learned the importance of technique. With gentle Christy, I learned that trust could make a difference. I would need that knowledge and much more when I moved to the utter chaos of day shift on the teen unit.

5. My Days with Teens

Teens had been rare when I was working on the medical unit and issues of embarrassment meant little when caring for children who regarded us as substitutes for their mommy and daddy. Dealing with issues surrounding dying had been at the center of my attention, and I learned to handle that well. I was, after all, working with staff who were very experienced at caring for dying children. But I was far from prepared for what I would face when I transferred to day shift working with teenagers. I expected, for instance, a steamy caldron of teen romance. I never saw a single one. Apparently, when teens are sick enough to be in a hospital, they don't feel romantic.

Instead, I discovered something quite different. Silly as it sounds, the best illustration of work on the teen unit was a cheap, molded plastic, 'work of art' that someone had placed in our snack room. It showed a little boy and girl turned so they were looking at the viewer but at the same time their naked buns were visible for all to see. That sort of exposure was true everywhere in the hospital, but somehow on the teen unit, with near-adults as patients, it seemed more vivid. That's one key to understanding how I came to write this book.

A Typical Day with Teens

Now is as good a place as any to explain what my typical day was like. Keep in mind that I was on a dedicated-to-teens (adolescent) unit at a nationally recognized children's hospital at a particular time and place. That meant we handled a disproportionate share of the more complex and difficult cases, hence all the terribly sad situations you'll read about here. Your situation may be different, particularly if you're mixed into the general population at a community hospital in a small town.

The unit was divided into three clusters centered on two multi-bed rooms, each holding either four girls or four boys and usually handled by a nurse/aide team. Around that pair of rooms were several private rooms for individual patients of either sex. The decision—undoubtedly a practical one—to mix boys and girls on each of the three clusters meant that there'd always be a gender mismatch between staff and patients. There wasn't a cluster for guys staffed by a male nursing staff—if such a thing were even possible. There wasn't a cluster just for girls.

As nursing staff, of course, we had to go in and out of rooms dealing with patients of both sexes, whatever their circumstances or state of undress. The result, thought of in terms of a potential for embarrassment, was a higgledy-piggledy situation in which the only rule was that the boys couldn't visit the girls rooms or vice-versa. The privacy of patients of one sex was at least protected from that of the other. If we didn't have that rule, I'm sure guys would have hung about the girls rooms for reasons other than conversation.

Beleaguered Guys

In that situation, the guys had it far worse. If a guy had any sense of modesty when he arrived, he had to get over it quickly. Most of their care was done by nurses, all of whom were women and many only a little older than they. Having aides alongside nurses didn't change the situation. Most were middle-age women coming back to work after having raised kids.

As I look back, the result was amusing—at least for someone who wasn't one of those unfortunate teen boys. Often confined to their beds and forced to wear those awful hospital gowns, they had no real privacy. At any time a female nurse or aide might dart up their bed, insisting that they do something they'd rather not do. As a result, I don't remember a single case where a conscious guy wasn't wearing the cotton briefs the hospital provided and staying carefully covered up with sheets. Pitiful as it was, that was all they could do to protect themselves from continual embarrassment.

So if you're a teen girl, feel sorry for those guys. They had it far worse than you. Their plight was so terrible, I couldn't begin to write a book about how they might deal with their embarrassments. If I wrote one, it'd be entitled *Hospital Nurses and Other Embarrassments* and would consist of two short sentences. "Give up. It's hopeless." Poor guys! I only hope that, by helping teen girls like you, this book also eases their plight.

Alas for me, that may be why, with two sets of exceptions, the guys I cared for seemed so sullen and withdrawn that all my efforts to get to know them came to naught. The exceptions explain the rule. The first exception was gregarious guys with major disabilities who'd long gotten over privacy issues and weren't playing male power games. The other exception was boys ten or eleven years old, who were little different from those I'd taken care of on Hem-Onc. After puberty, I decided, guys relate by determining who's the most powerful. When they're sick enough to be in a hospital, those power games don't work. An All-State quarterback may find himself in traction, completely dependent on a nurse to scratch his itching big toe. Not very macho.

Of course, I could have talked to these guys about how 'hot' their nurse was. There's a shallow type of male bonding in that. That wouldn't have been hard. Most of the unit's nurses were young, newly married, and quite pretty. I suspect that was because they valued evenings and nights home with their hubbies enough to endure the day shift's brutal work load, one of the worst in the hospital. But I couldn't talk about them that way. I knew those 'hot' nurses as friends. So most of the guys and I talked less than I wanted. My better relationships were with my nurses, as well as patients of the opposite sex.

Almost Private Girls

The girl's situation could not have been more different. Their privacy was almost complete. Their rooms were the domain of a nearly all-female nursing staff. That meant that they could be much more casual about their undress. Their situation was nothing like that for the guys.

I say "almost," because I was the one glaring exception. After I transferred, I discovered that I was the only male nursing staff on day shift—a bit like being the only guy at a girl's slumber party. If I'd known what I was getting into, I'm not sure I'd have taken the position. I soon realized that, if I wasn't going to ruin their slumber party and leave them as glum and trapped as the guys, I needed to earn their trust. So I adopted rules that I hoped would be obvious to them, the most important being that, although I couldn't avoid seeing that undress in my peripheral vision, I wouldn't look, much less stare. Most seemed to accept me on those terms.

Perhaps the best illustration of my dilemma is one I didn't realize at the time. Of all the hospital's staff, in my eyes the bravest were the medical technicians who did blood draws on younger children. When a new child was admitted, they were sometimes afraid of everyone on staff, but they quickly learned that aides in short tunics like me rarely did anything painful. When I came into their room, they'd smile.

But these kids also learned that those in long lab coats were usually there to do a painful 'poke.' The younger ones would scream loudly, squirm, and try to get away. Imagine spending much of your work day making kids terrified and miserable. It must have been awful. These medical technicians had to be very brave and often very caring—like the wonderful Elsie I'll mention later.

Working with teen girls could have been similar. Being a guy was like wearing a long lab coat. Remember Min. Something ordinary when a (female) nurse did it could have become embarrassing or even frightening for girls if it was done by me. It did no good for me to ignore the problem, even though that was how the hospital expected me to act. Nor could I avoid doing anything that might embarrass them. Like the medical technicians with their blood draws, these girls's routine care—including almost all the embarrassing stuff—was a part of my job. That meant that I could hurt some girls just as surely as the pokes those medical technicians administered. That's what I hated and what I fought against. Fixing that is what this book is all about.

Fortunately none of these girls would scream or cry when I came into their room. They were too old for that. In fact, taking into account their differing personalities, most of the time things went quite well. Min really was an exception. Almost all accepted and trusted me. That said, their varied views on what constituted embarrassment constantly astonished me. We'll be talking a lot about that.

Some were casual about it all, much like the Post-Op Girls I'll soon describe. I was more likely to get embarrassed than they. Others, those I call the Sensible Girls, were clever enough to keep what happened within their comfort zone. They're the ones who offer the best examples for you. In addition, there were girls like Heidi, Fay and Kay, who set firm guy rules, making clear what I could do and not do. With them I could relax, knowing I'd be put 'in my place.'

But that didn't mean there weren't complications. In their heart of hearts, all these teen girls had to decide if I could be trusted. In addition, some girls—particularly those we will get to know as Pala, Tina, Ginny, and Carina—were terribly vulnerable to being hurt by the practices at my hospital. Try though I might, it wasn't always easy for me to know what to do with such girls. You will discover why when I talk about them.

Our Shared Purposes

This book is about helping you cope with precisely those sorts of embarrassment problems. It will, I hope, make your hospital stay as free of embarrassment as possible. What are our shared purposes?

First, as the old saying goes, being forewarned is forearmed. I want you to acquire a feel for the unique world you'll be entering, so you'll be ready. Hospitals are like high schools in one respect. They have their own culture and their own, often unwritten, rules that you need to understand. Until you understand that culture, you'll thrash about, making mistakes. The experiences I'll be describing, varied as they are, should help you learn quickly.

Second, I want to free you to be yourself by showing you the wide range of options. You won't be in a position to police a room, making all the girls in it fit some standard of dress or undress. That's for the nurses to do, and in my experience that's a fairly loose standard. On the other hand, if you go along with the more casual girls, you may find yourself later asking yourself, once you get home, "Why did I let myself do that? That's not me." Your place in that continuum from casual to careful should be yours and yours alone. You don't have to behave like your roommates or the other girls you see. You can fit your hospital care to your comfort zone. Remember that.

Third, I want to offer concrete steps to make your hospital stay more enjoyable. As I'll point out later, quite a few common hospital practices could benefit from serious amending in how they're done, particularly with guys caring for teen girls. That said, for those guys who're bold enough to read a book that has "girl" in its title, much of what I say here should help you enjoy your hospital visit too. Behind what I say about dealing with embarrassment lies some helpful advice at taking better control of every aspect of your hospital stay and even your life.

Finally—and this is important—I believe that the issues I'll be discussing here aren't being neglected by hospitals because their staff as a whole are indifferent or cruel. That's not why most people go into medicine or nursing. Embarrassment issues really are secondary in comparison to the central importance of treating and healing patients, many with life-threatening illnesses like those you will meet in this book.

Since you've chosen to be in a hospital despite the risk of embarrassment, I imagine you feel the same. Dying or suffering from some serious sickness really is worse than being embarrassed. So remember that, if you were my patient and really sick, I'd be a lot more concerned about you dying or your sickness taking a turn for the worse than I would about embarrassment. Embarrassment really is secondary. That should be your attitude too.

That said, I also believe that secondary issues can interfere with medicine's primary goal of healing. In *Nights with Leukemia* I describe how administrative fault-finding turned staff against staff, endangering children. In this book I describe how an administrative obsession with work efficiency over all else has similar results. Curing patients should not come at the cost of emotional harm either to staff (as in *Nights*) or to patients like you (as here).

Next, we look in more detail at look at how I felt about this situation, drawing a comparison to how I felt about being forced to inflict pain on patients I liked. As you might guess, I don't like being a meanie.

6. Pain and Embarrassment

It happened while I was still on the medical unit. I knew from the start that this medical order was ridiculous. Gerry was about two and his vomiting was probably due to its most common cause, gastroenteritis, also known as the stomach flu. The resident on duty that night, however, thought otherwise, and ordered us to try different fluids, as if the little boy had suddenly developed an emotional, allergy-like reaction to one or two of them.

So I dutifully went through every liquid we had in the refrigerator—water, pedialyte, apple juice, orange juice, cranberry juice, and even milk. He threw up every one of them. By 1 a.m. the poor little boy was getting so thirsty, I discovered him trying to lick the vomit off his rubberized bed pad.

Enough was enough. The kid obviously needed an IV. I was so ticked off, I didn't bother with rank-conscious hospital protocol. I told the nurse what was happening and bluntly said, "Get the resident to order an IV." One was ordered and, a few minutes later, his thirst relieved, the little boy was sound asleep.

Choosing Both

Gerry's suffering and how quickly it was corrected once the problem was recognized illustrates why I felt so frustrated with embarrassment issues. I understood that medical care can be unpleasant. Working Hem-Onc put that in the starkest of terms. I cared for children getting dreadful chemotherapy drugs. I had to be with them in the middle of the night, holding a small bucket and trying to console them as they 'puked their guts out.' I hated that, but I learned to live with it. What we were giving them was good medicine—the best in the world. Without those drugs, their leukemia would kill them. If I couldn't cope with those complexities, I didn't belong on Hem-Onc.

I also understood the broader context. What I was facing is a common problem in hospitals. Medicine is often a choice not *between two evils* but instead *for two results*, one evil and one good. There's the pain and suffering that treatment may cause and that medical staff must inflict, and there are the benefits of the treatment, including hopefully a return to good health. We can't chose one or the other. We must choose both.

On a much smaller scale, Gerry's case illustrates that. Starting an IV on small children is painful and traumatic. They hate pokes. I know, I've helped nurses start them on untold numbers of kids. The resident may have meant well that night, hoping to avoid that trauma with his 'try many liquids' order. But as I told my nurse, no IV was going to be as bad as the thirst little Gerry was experiencing. He got over the IV poke within a minute. He'd have been miserable and awake all night with thirst. My frustration and anger rested in the fact that, due to a resident's initial bad judgment, we delayed what we should have done when the boy first arrived.

Embarrassment should have been handled more like that, with mistakes at least being followed by quick corrections. Like pain, it's a part of being in a hospital. Hospitals aren't elegant hotels. Staying in one often means strangers looking and touching in places where most patients don't want. Sickness and treatment also leave patients unable to do the things they normally do in private, making them dependent on others. That means bedpans, trips to the toilet, gown changes, and the like. That's just the way it is. Like pain, it's sometimes necessary.

Indifference and Silence

Unfortunately, embarrassment wasn't treated like pain and that's what irked me. We didn't talk about it as if it mattered. We didn't try to come up with ways to reduce the hurt it inflicts. Even when we were obviously getting it wrong, we didn't change what we were doing. Embarrassment was the problem that no one, me included, ever discussed.

I didn't come up with a way to reassure a frightened Min. When innocent little Maria made a whispered appeal to her nurse, she was quickly brushed onto me and, at the time, I acted no differently with her than I would have with a four-year-old boy. It didn't occur to me to take that nurse aside and say, "Listen, I think Maria asked you because she fears being embarrassed. She wants you to do it. I'm not trying to get out of work, but could you do this for her?" Remember, it was a slow night. Both the nurse and I had the time to do a bit extra.

And yes, a more assertive girl might have said to the nurse, "No, I want you to do it." Speaking up like that is big part of what I'll be teaching you. But the number of teen girls who can do that, especially just after arriving at a hospital, is vanishingly small. Most go along, even though they feel uncomfortable. That's what lay at the heart of my frustration. With pain we did the best we could. We anticipated how our patients might feel and made what corrections we could even without them asking. We almost never did that with embarrassment.

You saw that with Christy's end-of-life care. No nurse on Hem-Onc seemed to give a thought to any issues with a guy caring for a girl in her mid-teens who could do almost nothing for herself. And yes, those nurses knew and trusted me, but the real issue wasn't me. It was her and whether she would trust me. What mattered most—her feelings—simply weren't considered. Somehow, she and I managed to make it work. But it shouldn't have been up to just us. The system should have worked better than that.

It's also true that dealing with embarrassment can be much more complicated than dealing with pain. I know that all too well, and I suspect you do too. Pain is easy to predict. A poke with a needle hurts, and we flinch, grimace, or cry out. Embarrassment is not so clearcut or obvious. Some girls I cared for were so sensitive, it was almost impossible for me not to upset them. Others were so casual, they amazed me. Some I never figured out.

Let's put you in a typical situation. You're my patient and just had tummy surgery the day before. When I come up to your bed the next morning, I have two things in mind. First, as the surgeon had ordered, I need for you to 'cough and deep breathe,' so you'll be less likely to catch pneumonia and be stuck in the hospital for several extra days. Second, I needed to check your suture site for bleeding or infection.

The first is about pain and isn't that complicated. I know for certain that you'll find that first 'cough and deep breathe' terribly painful. That's why I try to make it a better by having you clasp a pillow tightly across your chest when you cough. Yes, in the end it still hurt a lot, but I'd done my best to make it better, and that helps you and I cope with my being a such meanie. Why did I know about that pillow trick? Because I'd been taught it. I was shown how to lessen pain.

The second of my tasks—checking that suture site on your tummy—isn't so clearcut. There, the issue is my embarrassing you—particularly if it's low on your tummy—and I have no way of knowing how you'll react to my peeking. Some girls will be happy with the attention and delighted to be told that the healing is going well. Others will be more Min-like. That meant that, as I came up to you, I couldn't know which you would be. Without intending, I could embarrass you and embarrassment also hurts.

Unfortunately, nothing I'd been taught helped when I had to peek under a gown like yours. There was no equivalent of clasping a pillow. In fact, the examples I saw were downright awful. A typical nurse could be brisk about that sort of thing. She'd rush up, yank down your sheets and flip your entire gown well up, so that everything imaginable showed. For her—assuming she was she—that was fine.

But if I'd done the same as a guy, I might have been exposing a bit more of you than you'd like. After a few fumbles—I hadn't taken care of many surgical patients on the medical unit—I learned to play it safe and carefully peal back only enough of the gown to see what I needed. That worked. No girl whose suture I checked ever gasped, glared, or became upset, much less slapped me. But why did I have to come up with that on my own? Why wasn't it taught?

As you will soon see, viewing sutures on girl's tummies was the least of the embarrassment issues I faced. As a result, I sometimes felt like a meanie (or worse), as I flailed about, trying to figure out what I'd never been taught—how to deal with embarrassment.

I think you get the point. I was frustrated, not because I couldn't give patients like you care that was totally free of pain and embarrassment. I knew that was impossible. I was frustrated because with embarrassment I didn't know how to do what I could to make girls like you more comfortable. I knew I could do better, but didn't know how.

Now we'll look at the first major embarrassment issue I faced after I began working with teen girls.

7. TRUSTING POST-OP GIRLS

Last year, I had surgery to fix an as-yet trouble-free hernia. As surgeries go, it wasn't much. I rode a night-owl bus downtown, walked a few blocks to the hospital, and arrived at the surgical unit at the appointed seven a.m. The surgery went well, and I was riding home with a friend by one that afternoon—something that would have amazed medicine a quarter-century ago. Because the only complications were four days of constipation and getting rid of ten pounds I could afford to lose, I was delighted to recover at home rather than in a hospital.

Since that was the closest I've ever been to hospitalization, I also gained some insight into myself as a patient. Afterward in the recovery area, a nurse brought me my clothes and drew a curtain that almost but not completely surrounded the area where I'd be dressing myself. At that point I thought, "What the heck. I don't care who sees. I just want to get out of here." Embarrassment was not the first of my priorities. Convenience was.

When I worked on the teen unit, I saw something similar. Some teens—even some of the beleaguered teen boys—had obviously decided that modesty was less important than convenience. Remember that when you're hospitalized. Although I'm doing my best to tell you how to avoid embarrassment, in some cases you may find that more trouble than it's worth. You may want to accept some intrusions and live with them. After all, convenience and comfort are important too. In other cases, despite all your well-intentioned efforts, you'll get embarrassed. Remember that's just part of being in a hospital. Laugh it off and move on. Life in too short to dwell on every little hiccup.

Summer Rush

Nothing illustrates choosing convenience over embarrassment better than an intriguing group I call the Post-Op Girls. When I first began working on the teen unit in the late spring, the staff was all abuzz about the coming summer rush. With school out, major surgeries on teens—ones that required weeks of flat-in-bed recovery—would begin. Many of these were spinal fusions that dealt with backbones that were twisting seriously out of normal. That sort of surgery was so much a speciality of our hospital, at that time it had "Orthopedic" in its name.

Some were boys. When the surgeries began, one boy impressed me more than any other. His spinal problem was so severe, surgeons warned that the corrective surgery had a 50/50 chance of leaving him paralyzed. He went bravely ahead. Afterward, I was delighted to be assigned the infection control for his halo traction. That was a metal ring around his head with screws driven into his skull, allowing his spine to be kept in constant traction, (pulled taunt), while he lay down or sat up in a wheelchair for many weeks. It sounds grimmer than it was, but he was still one gutsy guy.

But most of our spinal fusion surgeries were for girls—six out of seven by the statistics. Very quickly, they were among my favorite patients. Why? Because they were just were just the sort of patient I hoped I would be—courageous, patient and practical. I liked them.

Their courage was obvious. Spinal fusion is only resorted to when all other means to keep an increasingly distorted spine straight fail. At that time, it often meant opening up the entire length of their backbone, forcing an S-shaped backbone to be straight by any means short of dynamite, and then placing two long stainless steel rods alongside to ensure it stayed straight. Surgeons call that 'instrumenting' the backbone, but it's more than that. It's a radical rebuild that left these girls with a steel backbone for the rest of their lives. And yes, they had the surgery because the alternative was far worse, but that doesn't lessen their courage one bit. These were brave girls. I thought highly of them and felt they deserved the best care I could give.

With the exception of a couple of girls who were understandably grumpy, they were also remarkably patient. At that time, the surgeries often took six to eight hours and, before coming to us, they had spent a week or more in a special, post-op recovery area flat on their backs, dependent on nurses for everything. The impressively long sutures that ran the length of their backs were almost healed by the time they came to us, and that takes time.

With us, they needed still more patience. In our care, they could roll occasionally from side to side, but otherwise they had to remain flat on their backs, not sitting up or standing at all. Recovery after they went home meant still more restrictions during what would be a long summer. What they were having to endure was far worse than my brief hernia surgery. These girls were putting the patience in patient.

Finally, much like me during my day surgery, most of these girls tilted toward causal undress as more convenient. Guys can wear undies and use a urinal without any problem. For these girls, because they were flat on their backs, each time a bedpan was used, their panties had to be pulled down almost to their ankles by someone else and then pulled back up afterwards. With their long, forced bed rest, most had decided that was simply too much bother.

Woeful Undress

As you might expect, that created issues. One girl in that sort of undress for a couple of days until she could get up and about was easy to manage. I'd only been on the teen unit a couple of months, but I'd gotten used to that. But three or four such girls flat on their backs in the same four-bed room for a week or more made looking elsewhere far more complicated. There was too much to not see.

When I first began to care for these girls, I knew my trustworthiness would be tested by the strangest of standards. If their undies came back on, they'd judged me odd. If they didn't, they trusted me and the room could stay relaxed, unlike those sadly beleaguered boys rooms. It felt good to know they trusted me, although I sometimes wished they hadn't. At the time, it was difficult to sort out what I found so frustrating. The problem, I thought, was their woeful state of undress. If only I could start my shift by insisting that they all don undies, all would be well. But that would never do. If I'd tried, my nurse would have laughed and told me I couldn't do that. This was their room, and their undress was their affair.

Looking back, I can see I was wrong. The problem wasn't that there was nothing underneath their gowns. That could be managed with a little finesse and a bit of understanding on both our parts. The problem lay in the well-ingrained habits their nurses in the post-op unit two floors up had taught them before they came to us. There the nurses had been kept very busy caring for these girls. Infection after such a serious back surgery was a great risk, and the need for regular dressing changes was critical. Just after their surgery, these girls would be exhausted, in pain, and left groggy by their pain medications. In that context, what they were doing made sense.

Coming to the teen unit, however, their situation changed. In most cases their almost two-foot-long incision down the center of their back had healed enough that their dressings were gone, and there was little for a nurse to do. Their orders were to lie flat on their backs, with an occasional, brief roll to one side. Their care was little more than meals three times a day, linen changes every few days, and bedpans every few hours. All were my speciality, so I became their primary caregiver. Meals on trays were easy, linen changes were more complicated, and bedpans drove me batty.

I explore what happened in more detail in the next chapter. Keep in mind that it places the issue of hospital embarrassment in its starkest terms, so I hope you'll excuse just how 'explicit' it is. I must tell the story right. At the same time, you'll also get a chance to meet those oh-so-clever Sensible Girls. You can learn a lot from them.

8. Sensible Girls

Looking back, I find it easy to blame my woes with those Post-Op Girls on those highly efficient post-op nurses. For instance, they'd taught these girls a specific way of helping when bed linens were changed. Of course, there was nothing special about that. It was the standard technique that I'd been taught during orientation, and it's often done exactly the same today. A girl was to roll on to her right side while the sheet on the left side of the bed was replaced. Then she'd roll over the new and old sheets to the left side of her bed while the old sheet was removed and the new sheet tucked in. It was quick and efficient—just what hospital administrators like.

Linen Changes

The problem came when a Post-Op Girl and I unwittingly used the standard technique. I feel like a fool to say this, but remember she and I didn't know any better. We were both doing exactly what we'd been taught. She would roll on her right side, and her gown would flop open, showing her buns. For reasons, I never understood, most girls in that situation don't adjust their gowns. I'd then do what I'd been taught with

Hospital Gowns and Other Embarrassments

the sheets and go to the other side of the bed. There, she'd roll over, showing her buns yet again.

That was frustrating. I liked these girls and saw them as little sisters. I'm sure they were no more happy about this than I was. They trusted me with linen changes in the same way they trusted the surgeon who'd done their spinal fusions. They weren't delighted with either, but they knew that both the surgeon and I meant well. Facing all they had to face, that was enough. Like me after my hernia surgery, they just wanted to be done and go home.

Fortunately, I did find a partial answer to all that rolling from side to side. Quite soon, a nearby aide, bless her heart, picked up on my frustration and came over to help. With she and I on opposite sides of the bed, the work went faster, the embarrassment was cut in half, and these girls seemed more relaxed.

A couple of months later, however, I realized that the real problem lay with the linen-change technique the girls and I had been taught. Rolling might be easier, but it wasn't the only option. As I cared for other girls whose surgeries were less extensive, some showed me a better way. Call them the Sensible Girls because they differ from both the extremes I'll be describing here. Not trained in that fourth-floor post-op unit and possessing buckets of good girl sense, they would wiggle their way across the bed, staying on their backs, and taking care to hold down their gowns with fetching modesty.

That was much better. That I could actually watch with amusement. And when I changed their sheets, it was much more pleasant to look a girl in the eyes and talk with her than it was to try to hold a conversation with a trusting but still embarrassed girl who was on her side facing away. So, if you find yourself in a similar situation, you might adopt the cute bounce-and-wiggle technique rather than rolling like a log. It may not be official, but it works fine.

Bedpans and Babies

Linen changes were merely awkward. Bedpan placements were absolutely terrible, although for much the same reason. Those mischief-making post-op nurses had taught these Post-Op Girls to adopt a bedpan pose that had their knees pulled up and their legs spread wide in a 'deliver my baby' posture. They'd done that so often in post-op, and it'd become so natural, that they seemed unconcerned when I replaced those nurses. I tried to tell myself that, if that was OK with them, it should be fine with me. That didn't work. I liked these girls, and this seemed too much like pornography. I coped by making my placements lightning fast, which probably increased their trust in me. But I was still so frustrated at being forced into the role of an unwilling obstetrician that on one occasion I simply ran away.

A girl's mother and father had been visiting and were leaving when the girl asked me for a bedpan. It was late afternoon, and I was exhausted. Each time I did bedpans for these girls, bless their wonderful hearts, I ended up in a silent, five-minute debate with myself over whether I was a voyeur. That was nonsense. No voyeur would go to as much trouble as I was going to not see, much less not to remember. But there was no way I could stop that accusing voice. As tired as I was, I felt I wasn't up to that yet again. The girl had chosen me over her own mother, but I called her mother back to handle that pesky bedpan. Like I said, it was frustrating almost beyond belief.

Again, the solution was simple. I did have my technique wrong, as least for a guy working with such trusting girls. A month or so after the Post-Op Girls left, as I became more experienced with teen-girl care, I realized that I was no longer feeling frustrated about bedpan calls. It'd become just another task. When I asked myself why, I realized that the procedure had changed without my being aware.

Again, it was those Sensible Girls. The bed-bound girls I was now caring for had less elaborate surgeries, ones that didn't required a long stay with those mischievous post-op nurses. They'd not picked up bad habits and were showing good sense when I responded to their bedpan call. You can think of them as the practical-minded middle between the two extremes we'll be discussing. Chances are, they're what you'll decide to be after reading this book.

Sensible Moves

How, you may be asking, were the Sensible Girls different from the Post-Op Girls? First, most Sensible Girls wore their undies from the very start, like all good girls in a hospital should—at least when guys like me are around. Undies aren't that much trouble and, in a hospital, they're almost like being fully clothed. Think of them as a swimsuit. With them on, you're fully dressed and ready for anything. And yes, that sounds silly, but it is realistic given how little that pesky gown conceals. So it's better undies than nothing. Later, I'll give more details and suggest a third alternative.

Second and more important, these Sensible Girls had their bedpan posture right. Keep in mind one reason for my dilemma. Viewed from

Hospital Gowns and Other Embarrassments

the outside, a girl needing a bedpan placed was a wide expanse of cotton sheet and gown. Misplacing it—especially the centering—by little more than a couple of inches meant wet sheets and a linen change. That mean more trouble for me and a great deal of embarrassment for her. To get that positioning right, I had to look, at least very briefly, at where it was going. That's why those trusting Post-Op Girls put me in such a terrible bind. It was 'deliver my baby' or wet sheets.

The Sensible Girls were different. As I slid in the bedpan, they kept their legs together and their knees low, which concealed a lot and meant the bedpan could be slipped in from the side rather than the front. When their knees still down, I'd slip their undies down to their ankles beneath their gown, a technique you may remember I'd adopted after Maria. Then they'd adopt that knees-high, legs-spread position to actually use the bedpan. Reverse the process, and there's little or nothing embarrassing going on. That was a great improvement and left me feeling far less frustrated. Now done right, bedpans became just another task.

Unfortunately, many hospitals still teach that 'deliver my baby' pose as the one and only way to do bedpans. I suspect that's because the hospital administration, after consulting with pointed-headed experts holding digital stopwatches, have concluded that it is 3.4 seconds faster or something. (Faster because the girl doesn't have to change her posture.) But take my word for it, from an embarrassment point of view, the legs-low, knees-together technique is infinitely better and takes only a few seconds longer.

So if you get the chance, practice it beforehand at home with your mother, using a thick book as a substitute for a bedpan. View yourself as if you were in a movie and act like a professional actress. Get your moves right and experiment in advance with what you'll say to staff. Then politely insist on those moves when you're hospitalized. You might even use it with all the staff, so you're not singling out the guys. It might not be the most efficient way, but they won't mind. You might even get some to informally adopt this girl-tested way.

Keep in mind that almost all the teen girls I cared for were sensible and cooperative. I liked them. They wanted to be helpful rather than temperamental prima donnas. They were willing to be flexible and reasonable. What they didn't like were procedures that seemed almost deliberately designed to be embarrassing. I got along well with these Sensible Girls because I was flexible enough to let them take the lead with bedpans, and they taught me a better way. Even better would be a hospital where legs-low, knees-together is what guys are taught and expected to do. As I'll be saying over and over again, hospital administrators need to realize that male and female staff aren't quite interchangeable. Some adjustments should be made.

Those most impressive Sensible Girls are also why I'm optimistic that, were hospitals to adapt their techniques, all would go well. Hospital care won't grind to a stop as a staff woman has to be found for every girly need. Guys on staff would simply follow a slightly different procedure, teaching it to girls when necessary.

The Sun Is Shining Again

One final remark about those amiable Post-Op Girls. You may find yourself in a similar situation to theirs, one where you've had a successful treatment for something serious with few or no complications. The news in your life is good and the sun is shining again. Enjoy that, and perhaps take the chance to spread some cheer to staff and patients alike. There's a lot of sadness in hospitals you might help alleviate.

At the same time, don't let your exuberance or your desire to brush aside petty hassles lead you to be more casual than necessary, particularly around guys. Looking back, I appreciate the trust those lovely Post-Op girls put in me. It was kind of them, and I did see it as a great compliment. Their trust helped me handle other situations where things got a bit more complicated.

But I'd have really rather been treated as something other than an honorary female. I didn't mind changing how I did things for girls. I just needed help discovering how. Remember, at that point I'd spent almost all my time in the hospital caring for little kids. About the only modesty-enhancing technique I knew was to move quickly. Teen girls were a new experience, and I was floundering badly.

Also, keep in mind something humorous but true. As a guy, I couldn't do what any woman nurse could easily do. I couldn't ask these girls to let me to try several different bedpan techniques, one after the other, to discover what worked best. I had to muddle through with what I'd been taught, even when it was obviously flawed.

In the end, there are two kinds of trust in guy-with-girl situations at hospitals. One has the girl thinking, "I'm going along with this embarrassing thing, because I don't think you mean me any harm." That's how the Post-Op Girls treated me. They trusted me and for the most part relaxed. That's fine as far as it goes.

But there's a further level of trust that thinks, "I trust you to work with me to discover something we both find less intrusive and embarrassing." That's much better because it involves communication and cooperation. That's also one of the most important points in this book, so I'll be repeating it often. Don't be Miss Ever Shy. Speak up about what you want and politely insist on it. Later, I'll explain how you can do that and still be everyone's favorite patient.

In the chapters that follow, I'll describe some patients who could not be more different from either those Post-Op Girls or the Sensible Girls—girls I also found myself liking, although for much different reasons.

9. RULE-MAKING HEIDI

Heidi was one of my favorite patients. She had lots of spunk, something I admire. I still have two pictures of her. In them, she has lovely light-brown hair, beautiful eyes, and a terrific smile. But in both—one in a wheelchair and the other lying in bed—the large, S-shaped curve in her spine is all too obvious.

Heidi was a fighter. Her original problem wasn't with her spine. It was an abdominal tumor. What followed was a tragic chain of events. The one-sided radiation used to treat the tumor so damaged her back muscles on one side that her spine began to twist. At that time, her chances of defeating the cancer seemed so slight, she decided not to have a spinal fusion. Given what that involves, that's understandable.

But Heidi whipped her cancer, and was left with a slowly twisting spine. Unfortunately, by that point spinal surgery was impossible, and a back brace would do so little good, I never saw her wearing one. She'd gone from one bad to another. That cancer wouldn't kill her, but her increasing spinal curvature almost certainly would.

Teen Tragedies

Heidi's situation is the best place to step aside and mention something you should keep in mind as you read. That's the relationship of embarrassment to the larger issues that were the real center of my attention on both Hem-Onc and the teen unit.

On Hem-Onc the emotional issues were simple and direct. Within months the outcome was usually settled. Our children either relapsed and died or, if they lived, were cured to live almost normal lives. However sad I might be, their dying was not like my dying. Their childish understanding was too different from mine for me to identify with them. I didn't see myself as them. I saw myself as incredibly blessed that I had not had to face as a child the enormous burdens they faced.

On the teen unit, however, my emotional responses were more conflicted. Yes, I still cared for patients with cancer and could see that same clear line between living and dying. But I was also caring for a more complex mix of sickness and death. Some of my teen patients were in a terrifying limbo. What they had—for instance a severely curved spine (Heidi) or cystic fibrosis (the two girls I'll talk about next)—would almost certainly still kill them someday, but their dying was drawn out and unpredictable, with much suffering and many delays along the way. There was nothing simple about their lives or their pending deaths.

Even more unsettling, that distinction between them as patients and me as staff was far smaller. A teen like you is almost an adult, so their lives and understandings were like mine. For better and worse, I could identify with what they were going through much better than I could with a child. That reduced the emotional distance between us.

As I look back, there's something else that matters. At the time of the events in this book, I was roughly twenty years older the teens whose stories I'll be telling (mid-teens versus mid-thirties). And yet here I am many years later in excellent health, while so many of those you will read about here—including Heidi and the Twins—are almost certainly dead. That haunts me. They lived and I knew them. Now they're gone, and yet I live on. And no, I don't feel survivor guilt. I didn't survive the illnesses that killed them. I never had those illnesses.

What I do feel is a regret for what these teens did not get from us. True, the medical care that we gave was state of the art at that time. For instance, we were one of the first hospitals in the world to do bone marrow transplants on children and teens with leukemia, something that can save a life that would otherwise be lost.

But at another level we—me included—failed to treat them as well as we might. To put it simply, we were too purely medical. We failed to take as seriously as might the emotional content of their lives and the fear and loneliness of their struggles. In a few chapters I'll be describing a fourteen-year-old girl named Pala, newly diagnosed with leukemia. She was my patient, and yet little that I'd been taught prepared me to treat her terrible plight any differently from someone who was in for a minor surgery. That wasn't good and that still bothers me.

Today's hospitals, particularly cancer wards in children's hospitals, seem much better at handling the complex emotions that go with sickness and death. But unfortunately, I can't see evidence that embarrassment, privacy and violation are being dealt with much better now than then. That's one reason for this book. It's intended to start a much-needed conversation.

Heidi's Rules

Now back to feisty Heidi. When they're at home, patients with limited mobility often have trouble getting about and making new friends. So when they were with us, they were often very sociable, seeing their visit as a great way to meet people. That's why Heidi would be up, dressed and getting about in her wheelchair, while many healthier patients were still in bed wearing their gowns.

In that getting up and dressed lies a story. Many of those with major disabilities could not dress themselves, and some required two people, their nurse and I, to help. Heidi was like that, but I was never asked to help dress her—not once. She had rules about that sort of thing. I also knew that, if I responded to her call light and she asked for a bedpan, she meant for me to get the nurse.

Yes, the hospital might be a little muddled in its thinking about guys with girls, but Heidi wasn't. Her mind was clear. I was a guy and she was a girl. That meant I must to stay in my place, which was nowhere nearby when she was dressing. I could take her temperature and bring her a lunch tray. I did that every day. I could certainly talk with her when I had the time. We did a lot of that. But nothing more personal than that. Even more important, Heidi didn't personalize her rules. She didn't have any problems with me as a guy and did not treat me as evil. She simply thought I had no business dressing her, which is reasonable.

I liked that. From my perspective, the teen unit suffered from a woeful lack of guidelines about what a guy like me should be doing—or at least how I should be doing it. The Post-Op Girls trusted me and were happy with my care. The Sensible Girls showed me how to do that care better. I also learned from girls like Heidi who made strict rules about guys. Even in all my confusion, I suspected that her unwillingness to accept guy-with-girl embarrassment hinted at what many less strong-willed girls were feeling or might soon feel once they got over their initial shock. They wanted to set rules but didn't know how.

That's why this book tells you how to be like Heidi and make rules of your own. The good news is that I never heard anyone on staff complain about the additional work such girls created—typically nurses doing bedpans and dressing them. The same should be true of you. The bad news is that, if you do nothing, nothing will happen. I'll say more about that later.

Odd as it sounds, once I settled in on the teen unit and learned the basics of caring for teen girls, I felt equally comfortable caring for girls at both extremes. The Post-Op Girls trusted me enough, there was little risk I'd do something that'd embarrass them. At the opposite extreme, Heidi set such clear rules, as long as I stayed within her limits, all went well. And given that they knew what they wanted, I also got along well with the Sensible Girls. Since those three groups made up the majority of my patients, my initial frustrations began to fade a little after my first summer. I began to make fewer blunders.

But that doesn't mean that there weren't some most serious problems with some girls. We'll take them up just after looking at when it makes sense for you to speak up about your care.

10. Speaking Up

It was early afternoon and, as I walked past this fifteen-year-old girl's room, I heard her coughing a peculiar, tickle-in-my-throat sort of cough that I'd heard before on Hem-Onc. "It sounds like she's getting air in her central line," I thought. I rushed into her room and checked the clear plastic tubing near where it entered a large vein just below her shoulder blades. No doubt about it—it was air. In seconds, a bubble of that air could reach her heart or brain, triggering a heart attack, a stroke, or even death. Air in a central line is rare but very dangerous.

I knew what to do. Moving quickly, at the same time I switched off her IV pump with my right hand, slipped the pillow out from under her head with my left, and asked her to turn on her left side, keeping her head low. Hopefully that would keep those deadly air bubbles in her lungs where they'd do much less harm. If one of those bubbles reached the right side of her heart, it would be only inches away from her brain by a major artery.

Doing as Told

That story illustrates an important point. In a hospital, sometimes the best thing to do is exactly what staff tell you and as quickly as possible. That can save your life or prevent serious injury. This was one of those cases. Her quick response to what I said made a difference. It wasn't a time to ask why I was giving those orders.

But that 'patients should do as staff tell them' rule also has downsides. Some are funny. From what I've read, men in nursing situations like to tease patients to encourage them to lighten up and relax. I know I tried that, but my well-meant teasing often drew a blank.

For instance, some girls liked to read *Seventeen* magazine. Knowing that a particular girl was sixteen, I'd tell her that the hospital didn't permit that, that only seventeen-year-olds were allowed to read it. Rather than get the point—that I was being silly and laugh—a girl would look at me with a strange expression, as if she didn't know what to do with what I'd just said. Over time, as similar attempts at gentle teasing fell flat, I came to realize that my teasing skills were woefully lacking. Used to doing precisely what I said—as all good patients think they ought—these girls didn't know how to respond when what I said was ridiculous.

Explaining What You Need

In other situations, this top-down structure, where staff gave the orders and patients quietly obeyed, created problems. On the teen unit, one came when a sick patient became well enough to get up and use a toilet rather than sit uncomfortably on a bedpan. That was good news and often a sign they'd be going home soon. But it also created issues. To keep someone who's stiff and wobbly from falling down, I had strict orders to give them all the help they needed getting to and from the toilet. That was a rule that must be followed. I'd be in big trouble if one of my patients fell.

Teen guys were easy, although some were so large I wondered if I'd be of any use if they began to fall. My biggest problem came with deciding just how much assistance a teen girl required. Walking them to our in-room toilet was obviously necessary. If they slipped walking on the slippery linoleum floor in socks, they could hurt themselves. But how much further should I go? Should I just take them to the door and trust them to handle the rest? That was an easy cop out. The room was small, hardly big enough to turn around in, and had sturdy handrails all around. Inside, falling was much less likely.

But some of these girls were extremely sick. They might take a minute or more just to stand beside their beds. Some had juvenile arthritis severe enough that every move was slow and stiff. Some had strokes that had left them partly paralyzed. Some were recovering from major surgeries that made bending at the waist extremely painful. Others were befuddled from pain medications. That's why it often seemed both kindest and safest for me to help them onto the toilet at the expense of a little embarrassment.

But how did I draw the line between helping and not helping? I ended up using my own judgment and fortunately that worked. The girls I helped seemed to appreciate my assistance. No one I left to her own skills ever slipped and fell. Unlike my woeful attempts at teasing, I had a knack for understanding a patient's limitations.

That knack did create problems with my nurses though. Some of those I worked with took chances with patients to save time. Others were careful almost to a fault. Both had default rules that valued either speed or safety. At times, I clashed with both, because I did my best to decide based on the patients themselves.

To use an example I will describe in more detail later, when I needed to leave Pala to get a change of clothing for her, I asked myself, "If I tell her, will she remain lying down?" I felt the answer was yes, so that's what I did. I did not trust other patients to follow similar instructions. Something inside told me that was wisest. That meant that at times I might seem to take big risks with patients, leaving them in a tub for instance, while with others I'd watch them like a hawk. It all depended on how I 'read' a particular patient. And I seemed to get it right. During over two years at the hospital, no patient I cared for was ever injured by my neglect.

But not all staff had that knack. That's where you enter this story. When situations like walks to the toilet arise, don't be afraid to speak up. You know what you can do better than anyone else. As you approach the toilet, either say: "I'm so sore and stiff, you'll need to help me sit down." or, "I can handle it from here myself." And yes, what you're saying has to be subject to at least one staff veto. If you're groggy from drugs, your judgment could be flawed. Painkillers can really addle your mind.

Notice that, by doing that, you're not being an insubordinate or bossy patient. From my perspective, what you've just done is great—enough I'd like to give you a little hug as you and I walk ever so slowly along.

Hospital Gowns and Other Embarrassments

Yes, judging by how a girl stood up and walked, it wasn't hard to decide how easily she could sit down. But judging how she would feel about being embarrassed was much more difficult, particularly for a new patient. That's why telling me (meaning that guy staff) what you'd like helps both of us. You know better than I if you want convenience and safety, meaning help, or modesty with a little grimacing and pain.

Also, keep in mind that this isn't just a guy-with-girl issue. Women on staff can benefit from your guidance. You may need to tell a speed-demon nurse that you're not in that great a shape and need her help all the way to sitting down, otherwise, she'll disappear at the door. And you may need to tell a safety-first nurse that she needn't worry, that you can take care of yourself despite her fretting. She probably has a lot to do.

Did you catch that? I'm giving you one of the most important lessons I have to offer. Yes, for the medical problem that brought you to the hospital and for emergencies like air in a central line, it's wisest to do what you're told. You're not a surgeon, so rely on a surgeon's expertise for the cutting stuff. But for a lot that happens in a hospital—particularly issues involving comfort and embarrassment—you're the real expert and should speak up. I'll be stressing that over and over.

Next, we'll look at two girls who did not hesitate to make their views known to me.

11. Normal Fay and Kay

Alas, there were two other girls who, unlike Heidi, did have major problems with the fact that I was a guy. I'll call them the Twins because, although they weren't related, they were often in at the same time and assigned to adjacent beds in the same room. Both had cystic fibrosis, and that matters a lot.

Girls with an Attitude

It was obvious to me that the Twins had an attitude problem. Often in for a week or more at a time for a 'tune-up,' they weren't happy when staffing assignments made them my patients. If fact, I got the distinct impression that they would have liked to have a sign at the entrance to their room: "Women Only. All Men Will Be Shot on Sight." As a certified, card-carrying male, I was a *persona non grata* in their eyes.

Why were the Post-Op Girls happy with me caring for them in spite of their undress and dependence, while the Twins resented my very presence even though they never needed my help with anything private? At first glance, that makes no sense.

Looking back, I suspect the reason lies in the differing life stories of the two, and especially the radically different futures each now had. A few months before, the lives of both would have seemed similar. Both faced a future clouded with uncertainty, with early death a distinct possibility. Both were being denied what many teens value above all else, a sense of normalcy. Neither could live the usual life of a teen. Neither could be certain of living as long as their friends.

For the Post-Op Girls, their future could have been like that of Heidi, severe disability followed by death as the curvature of their spines increased, crushing their vital organs. The Twins faced an equally bleak future. They were part of a cystic fibrosis generation that had lived longer than any previous one, but one that still faced a drastically shortened lifespan.

Suddenly the life paths of these two diverged. Their surgeries successful, the Post-Op Girls could look forward to a bright future. They didn't need to grasp at illusions of normalcy. They had it, full and abundant, perhaps for the first time since their early teens. While I was researching what I would write about them, I came across a video of a girl who'd recovered from a spinal fusion and become a cheerleader. She was doing flips I'd never dare with my completely normal back. Except for the fact that they'd set metal detectors at airports ringing wildly, these Post-Op Girls were now like other girls their age.

That may be why they didn't mind having me around. I wasn't an intrusion. Instead, I was a hint that they were returning to a normal world with fathers, brothers, guy classmates, and perhaps even a boyfriend. My guyishness in their hospital room signaled better to come. I brought normalcy. Even though I was a guy at their slumber party, I was a welcome guest.

Sadly, no such good news awaited the Twins. Their desire for normalcy was as great as that of the Post-Op Girls, but it was being cruelly denied. No surgery could cure the many and complicated problems that cystic fibrosis creates.

That was the situation when I blundered into their lives. It's not normal to have a strange guy coming into your bedroom before you've dressed in the morning and insisting on taking your temperature (under an arm), looking at your chest (respiration), and holding your hand (pulse). In fact, it's downright weird. They were right to regard me as an intrusion. That's what I was.

Fay and Kay

I'll now call the Twins Fay and Kay. Both were fighters, and both were survivors. As one of their doctors told me, the ones who live the longest with cystic fibrosis were those who refuse to let their disease dictate their lives. They fight desperately to be like others their age.

That was certainly true of these two. Both were in their early twenties, and both were part of a new generation that, at that time, was creating a stir in medicine. In the past, those with cystic fibrosis died young. My cousin died of it when she was about four. But some were now living well into adulthood. It no longer made sense to care for them in a children's hospital. Something else had to be found.

There's also a powerful emotional factor that didn't occur to me at the time. Keeping the Twins alive required a steady round of treatments and repeated hospitalizations—that tune-up I mentioned. Only as I wrote this, did I remember what that includes. One problem cystic fibrosis creates is that the mucus in their lungs is thicker than normal. Breaking it free requires hundreds of hard, daily 'claps' on their chest and backs by physical therapists. Since this was a hospital, Fay and Kay would have no choice about whether their therapist for the day was a guy or not.

Understanding that helps me to see why they saw me as a nuisance. They couldn't keep guy therapists from clapping their bare chests. Their lives depended on that. But they could shove me away, because they didn't need me. And if rejecting me helped them cope with their many hassles and made their lives seem more normal, I didn't mind.

A Desire for Normalcy

In fact, the desire of Fay and Kay for normalcy was so obvious, even their disdain for my presence didn't keep me from liking their sheer girlishness. Even if they could easily get up and about, most of our teen girls and boys would lounge in bed wearing their gowns until about ten a.m. Fay and Kay were up and dressed early, sometimes even before I arrived at seven a.m. They weren't sick. No, not them! They didn't need to be in bed or dress like someone who was unhealthy. No way! And when they got up, they didn't dress in Hospital Casual, meaning the baggy jeans and ugly, washed-too-often cotton tops the hospital provided. Instead, they were stylishly dressed in clothes they'd brought from home. They could have slipped out of the hospital and gone shopping at a nearby mall if they'd wanted. Again normalcy.

Fay's concern with her privacy even triggered the only such issue that came up during my over two years at the hospital. One of my patients was a girl with severe juvenile arthritis who needed assistance getting to the toilet. I walked her there and placed a basin we called a 'hat' in the toilet because there were orders to track her urine volume. Then I helped her inside, closed the door, and left her alone. When she finished, I walked her back to her bed and helped her get in. After that, I returned to the toilet to check her urine volume. When I opened the door, there was a scream of outrage. Fay must have needed to go really badly. In the maybe thirty seconds I'd been gone, she'd slipped into the toilet, removed the hat and sat down. She complained to the head nurse, but when I explained what happened, for once the head nurse understood.

I still have a picture of the other girl, Kay, chatting with a nurse. Her desire for normalcy was even greater than Fay's. During my roughly ten months of caring for teens, she was the only girl who took the time to make herself up each morning and the result—a most pretty girl—is obvious in the picture. Normal teen girls know their makeup, and no hospital stay was going to change that for her. Normalcy, almost in excess.

Ponder for a long moment the plight Kay was in as a girl interested in guys. How would you feel if you had to tell a boy who's starting to like you, "I've got cystic fibrosis. You don't really want to fall for me. I could die at any time." Most of us don't know how good we have it.

Sadly, all Kay's desperate attempts at normalcy couldn't give her the good health denied her from birth. She contracted a lung infection that our antibiotics could not whip and died a few days later in the ICU. Her long struggle for normalcy was over.

Kay illustrates why I never minded being on the wrong side of a patient's bad moods. Most had so much going on in their lives—so many burdens to bear and pains to suffer—it wasn't fair for me to expect them to be perfect. The minor hassles they imposed on me were nothing compared to the troubles they faced each and every day. You might remember that if one of your fellow patients is difficult to be around.

A Darkening Future

Like the Post-Op Girls, the Twins offer a lesson you might take to heart. Your attitude toward the future may shape how you deal with the demands of a hospital. If that future is good, you may respond one way.

If it's bad, you may react differently. I've already mentioned a brightening future. Now I'll talk about the opposite.

If your life is constricting, with fewer choices open and treatment demands you hate, you're likely to grasp at any feeling of control that's available, even if it doesn't make sense. Like the anger Christy's mother had toward her daughter's nurses, that can lead you to be cold toward those on staff who mean you no harm and can even cause you to resent normal hospital activities. That's not good.

It's true that getting cold-shouldered by the Twins was something I could live with. I knew enough to make allowances. But I'd have still rather not have been treated like a guy who might, at any given moment, hurl one of them onto a bed and rip her clothes off. And yes, that's roughly what their physical therapy involved, but it wasn't something I'd ever do. I liked them, and my job wasn't intrusive in the slightest. I took their vital signs once a shift, I brought them their meals twice each day, and I changed their sheets when they were out of bed. They had no reason to see me as an enemy.

So if you find yourself in a similar situation, recognize where you're coming from and realize that guy probably means well. Treat him kindly and even offer an apology when one is deserved. We can't help being guys. We're just born that way. You might even find that the guy you're seeing as an intrusion might be worth getting to know. I'd have certainly liked to have known Fay and Kay a little better, perhaps to make up for losing that cousin of mine who died so young from cystic fibrosis.

You might also want to learn something else from the hospital-savvy Fay and Kay. Don't let sickness control your life or force any more dependence on you than absolutely necessary. Fight for normalcy. As soon as you can, get up and walk about. Abandon that pesky bedpan and use the toilet as soon as possible. Dress in a way that pleases you. We never minded helping a patient get up and about, even though that meant more work. We were there to get them well. More activity meant a patient was getting well and going home. That was good.

So if you like, as soon a your nurse says it's OK, get rid of that dreadful hospital gown and dress in your best street clothes. Just think through which clothes are best. When you're still stiff and sore from surgery, a tight pair of jeans might not be the best choice.

Next, I'll explain why you may have an easier time bringing up a touchy topic than the seemingly more experienced people who care for you. Staff have more trouble knowing what to say than you realize.

12. Saying It Wrong

For reasons that made little sense, I often felt a special responsibility for patients I admitted to the unit. Technically, all I did was ask them a few questions and give them a small yellow bin filled with things like soap and toothpaste. But when I did that, something clicked in my head that left me feeling like I'd now become personally responsible for everything that happened during their stay. It was almost like, by doing the admission paperwork, I'd ordered their admission to the hospital. Yes, that seems crazy, but life is often crazy.

Kate's Heart Surgery

Kate was one of my admissions. She was in her early twenties and had spent much of her life having surgeries to correct various heart defects. Now almost too old for a children's hospital, she was in for yet another one. I admitted her late one afternoon and the following morning she went for her operation. Heart surgery is serious, so when it was over she went to the ICU rather than back to us.

About a week later, she returned to us, her arrival shrouded in guilt and mystery. Something had gone badly wrong post-op. An IV with sodium bicarbonate had leaked into the tissues of her arm, with a result that Drugs.com describes grimly: "Inadvertent extravasation of intravenously administered hypertonic solutions of Sodium Bicarbonate have been reported to cause chemical cellulitis because of their alkalinity, with tissue necrosis, ulceration or sloughing at the site of infiltration."

"Tissue necrosis" means the death of tissue, in her case the muscles of her lower right arm, which was now a sickly looking pale grey. It was one of the most depressing sights I experienced, worse even than the exit wound of a boy's shotgun accident. The latter left a crater so large, I could almost stick my fist inside.

A few days later, when it came time for Kate to go home, I took her mother and her, in the obligatory wheelchair, down to their car. Their visit hadn't been a pleasant one, so there was a coldness surrounding them that I foolishly tried to ease by remarking that they probably wanted "to blow this place up."

That was not a good move, and neither said a word. My blunder does, however, illustrate the point I want to make here. As staff, it's often hard for us to know what to say in difficult situations. Typically, we don't know patients that well, so what we say often goes wrong. That's particularly true with embarrassment.

Not So Witty Me

As I wrote this book and its two companion volumes, I often thought of situations that could have been better handled if I'd only said something brilliant and witty to a patient much like you. That still bothers me, and I mention some of those 'I should have said' situations. But it's also true that much of the time, it was best for me to simply do my job, showing I cared by what I did. Words might have created problems.

Gentle Christy, the girl who died on her fifteenth birthday, is an example of that. Her family life was so filled with conflict, it was hard for me to know what to say. So I focused on giving her the best care I could and making her nights as peaceful and comfortable as possible. More than that would have been too much. I simply didn't know how to make small talk with her. It was too risky.

If that's true with dying, it's also true for the chief theme of this book—embarrassment. Yes, it might have helped a girl if I said something to ease an embarrassing situation. But that was fraught with a risk that, not knowing the girl, I might say something wrong. I might try to be humorous or teasing, when she might not be in a mood to appreciate that. I might treat the matter with great seriousness, when she'd have rather it just be over and done with. And I was always aware that simply talking about something could make it more obvious and thus worse. Often, it seemed better to pretend nothing was happening.

Yes, to some extent, I treated such situations like I would removing tape or a bandaid. Sometimes simply yanking a bandaid off in one quick and smooth move was best. The pain was so brief, it was easily forgotten. Embarrassment can be like that. The quicker the better, as with those Post-Op Girl bedpans.

At other times, quickness wasn't possible There was no way to quickly help Jennie, the girl with juvenile arthritis I mention later, into a bathtub. She had to move slowly and carefully. On an occasion like that, small talk did work. I'd talk about anything trivial that came to my mind. Saying nothing of importance eased the situation and didn't bring up the risk of saying something stupid.

You Are Different

But keep in mind that your perspective is different from mine. As staff, I was expected to be flexible and patient. I knew how to handle all sorts of moods. I was healthy, not in pain or facing a terrible future, nor was I the one facing embarrassment. That means I was easy to talk with. So if you'd been my patient, you could relax and say whatever came to your mind. I would not get upset. Whatever you might think to the contrary, you could lead our conversation much better than I could.

Yes, amazing as it sounds, your jokes are not going to fall flat. If joking about something painful or embarrassing helps you to get through it, go ahead with my blessing. And if you tease me, I won't take it wrongly. I'll be charmed that you're so relaxed. Most staff like talking with patients. It beats the boredom of doing the same thing day after day.

You also have other options. What you see as frivolous and fun, I'll take as the same and laugh with you. What you regard as serious, I'll regard it as serious too. Even if you get ticked off and call me a "blundering, clumsy oaf," I'll tell myself that, next time, I should not be so awkward. I can learn much more from direct criticism than from a cold stare.

In short, while I need to be careful with what I say to you, as a patient you can feel speak freely with me or others on staff. I know you may not feel that way, wondering perhaps if we might get mad and punish you. ("No pain meds for you today, girl. You insulted me with that silly comment.") But that isn't true. We're used to dealing with all sorts of people and can adjust easily. If saying something helps, then say it.

This isn't just about embarrassment either. Speaking up eases a lot of situations. If a new nurse seems nervous about starting an IV, say something to lighten her mood. You'll not only make her day a bit better, by helping her to relax you're helping her get that IV started on the first try. That you should like.

I think you get the point. Hospital staff aren't machines. Most appreciate talking with you. It helps lighten their daily grind. By talking with us in a relaxed and free way, you can help us do our jobs and better understand how to care for you. Remember, we're not mind readers. If you want something, you need to ask for it.

Now, I'm going to shift from generalities to something intensely practical. I'll be talking about bedpans and the almost soap-opera politics that surround them. Understanding why hospital staff do what they do will make it easier for you to steer what happens in directions you like.

13. YOUR BLUSHING TOES

From time to time, I'd have two girls in adjacent beds who should have been calling on me for bedpans about equally often. The first would ask every few hours. The other never did, despite the fact that I was constantly in and out of their room. I sometimes joked to myself that the second, who was often quite friendly, either had a bladder the size of an oil drum, or she was being careful to wait for situations when only a nurse was in the room. Then she'd ask for help in a direct way, perhaps saying something like "I *really* would like it if *you* would get my bedpan?" Most nurses are kind and, even if they're feeling rushed, hunting up me would take longer than doing it herself. That second girl got the privacy she wanted. The first got me, which since she could see what the other girl was doing, must have been OK with her.

That 'wait for the woman' technique—one that by its very nature I never saw—illustrates what you should do if you have a guy on staff caring for you and you rather not have some things done by him. But to do it right, there are some things that you should keep in mind. Here I assume, as in my case, that she's a nurse and he's an assistant. Adjust to fit your situation.

First, planning is everything. If you wait until you absolutely have to go, the nurse may not appear as you wiggle, squirm and cross your legs, feeling like you're about to die. "Should I hit the call button?," you wonder. That will mean someone will come, but, as luck would have it, it's likely to be the guy. If the nurse is on break or at lunch, asking him to get her will get you nowhere. So the first rule is to plan ahead. Don't wait until you absolutely have to go. That may be too late. Go when you can go. Keep that bladder of yours well below the bursting point.

Second, keep in mind that, despite your most fervent hope, the woman who's caring for you can't read your mind. In fact, when she's busy—which is most of the time—she simply doesn't have the energy to try. She has lots to do, and, if bedpans are part of that guy's responsibilities, she expects him to handle them. Remember what I told you about Maria when she asked the nurse for a bedpan? That's your situation. If you want things to be different, you're going to have to make them different. You'll have to speak up and ask in the right way.

Third, show some sympathy for the guy. In all probability, he doesn't want you either groaning with pain or embarrassed. He's as trapped by the system as you are. Hospitals are very task-oriented. Everyone has a job they're expected to do. Nurses do medications, while assistants do the more manual tasks, such as food trays, linen changes, and bedpans. There's hardly enough time for each to do what's already expected of them. Any work the nurse has to pick up makes her already hard day even worse.

The Problem with Tasks

In my case, that task-oriented division of labor put me in a bind I hated. I'd have loved to have been able to tell every bed-bound girl that I'd handle her private needs as quickly and with as little embarrassment as possible, but that, if she had a problem with that, I'd be happy to get the nurse. Unfortunately, that'd be promising more than I could deliver. A few of the nurses I worked with were so marvelously kind, they wouldn't have complained. But most would insist that, by making such a blanket promise, I was dumping work on them. There would have been a conversation with the head nurse, and my 'get a nurse instead' offer would be utterly banned. The situation would get worse rather than better.

So, instead of a blanket promise made to all, I evaded a policy I thought sometimes cruel by cheating carefully. I reserved that 'get a nurse instead' offer for special situations. With Christy, who was dying of a brain tumor, if she'd asked me for a nurse, I could have stressed to the nurse the terrible situation she was in. With shy girls, I would turn their meekly whispered request for a nurse into a much more assertive insistence. I'd make them roar like a lioness with, "The girl in Bed 3 needs to see you as soon as possible." I didn't have to say that I knew it was just for a bedpan. They'd find that out for themselves.

Keep in mind that even the best-hearted of staff can't do everything you might want. If you were my patient, you could be sure that, if some crisis developed, something that perhaps only I could see and that might threaten your life, I'd do everything in my power to get you the care you needed, even if it meant putting my job on the line. And in a situation like that of Pala in the next chapter, one where I must brave a nasty administrative attack to protect your feelings, I'd do it gladly.

But most hospital care isn't like that. Most embarrassment issues are more like preferences. You'd rather a woman take care of something rather than a man, but you don't see the latter as the end of the world, particularly since I've been showing you how to make it better. In those cases, if you were my patient, you'd find yourself playing second fiddle to the nurse. Yes, unfortunately, I'd be a bit more concerned about her feelings than yours. Why?

It's not because I want to be mean. It's because I must be practical. You're likely to be my patient for just a few days, and that matters. The nurse is someone I must work with day after day, week after week. I can't ignore what she thinks. Yes, it's selfish, but if I get her ticked off, it'll cause me more grief for far longer than your brief frustration with me will. That's why I needed to be careful about referring things like bedpans to her. After all, she can't refer IV antibiotics to me.

I'll let you in on a deep, dark secret, one that I wish weren't true. At my hospital—behind that unspoken and absurd hospital policy that male and female staff were identical—lay a pattern of intimidation directed at our teen patients, both guys and girls.

When I first began to work days on the teen unit, I expected get called every time a guy somewhere on the unit complained that he didn't want a blankity-blank woman changing his poop-filled diaper. (Yes, ugh!) After all, as a guy, I could understand why he might feel that way. But during my ten months of working with teens, I was never called to another cluster to deal with a guy's embarrassment issues. Their intimidation was so complete, they'd given up resisting and withdrawn beneath tightly drawn sheets. That's sad, so be glad you're a girl. You do get a bit more sympathy.

A Girl's Special Request

Judging by the staffing, our teen girls should have had it much better. After all, I was the only guy among the unit's six to eight daytime nursing staff. It might have made no sense for me to dash about, dealing with every guy-patient embarrassment issue on the entire 34-bed unit. If I did, I wouldn't have time for my own work. But with so many more staff women available, couldn't the hospital have been a bit more accommodating for girls? Dealing with the girl-see-guy issue might be impossible. But why weren't guy-see-girl issues dealt with more generously? Why were these girls always expected to deal with me and me alone?

Workflow and efficiency were why. Both my nurse and I circulated among 10 to 12 patients. If a girl or guy needed a bedpan or urinal, they could ask us as we passed through their room. The entire process might take about fifteen seconds twice, with the gap between filled by whatever had brought us into the room in the first place. That's efficient, and hospitals worship efficiency.

Compare that to a typical "special request." I enter your room to check the surgical dressing on one of your roommates, and your poor little bladder is about to explode into a million pieces. You are in agony, and I'm your only hope. You've waited and waited for the nurse, like I suggested earlier, but she's yet to show because—unknown to you—she's at lunch. I'm new to you and a guy with a beard (a little scary) and a kola bear on his stethoscope (more reassuring). But you're not sure if you can trust me. I might handle your bedpan like a nurse the day before did—the one who yanked down your sheets, flipped up your gown and, with the late afternoon sun pouring in the window, pulled your panties down to your blushing toes. So you marshall every bit of will power you have and ask me to get a female staff to deal with your bedpan.

I don't have a problem with that. I'd be happy to do as you want. But keep in mind what that special request means. Your nurse is gone, so I'm running the cluster all by myself. I'm very busy. To deal with what you've asked, I'll have to go to another cluster, find a nurse or assistant who doesn't look too harried, and plead with her to handle your needs, perhaps at the same time obliging myself to pay her a favor later. Remember, you're not only not her patient, if she's a nurse, doing bedpans isn't even her job. You're a double intrusion into an already demanding workload. That doesn't make staff happy.

Then there's the math. Thanks to your special request, thirty seconds of work by one person has turned into a several minute interruption in the work of two people. For a hospital, that sort of waste in unacceptable, so they reduce it to an absolute minimum with a grim form of silent intimidation that you may sense during your stay. They make it hard for you to ask for special treatment, particularly if your reason is girlish shyness, modesty or embarrassment. That creates a terrible 'Catch 22'—look up the term if you don't know its meaning. To have their special requests granted, girls must speak up. But girls who're embarrassed easily are also likely to be girls who're usually too embarrassed to speak up. They can't win for losing. It's not fair or kind. In fact, it stinks.

Asking a Favor

I will offer one ray of hope. A special request is hard on staff because it looks like a demand and usually comes at the wrong time. Asking for a favor in advance should work much better, especially if you add "whenever possible." It's not perfect, because it leaves a way out, but it's likely to be better received.

For instance, you might catch the nurse when she doesn't seem overwhelmed with work. Then say something like, "I'm rather shy [or easily embarrassed]. I wonder if, whenever possible, you could take care of my bedpan [or other embarrassing thing].... but only when it's convenient for you." You've given her a reason and some encouragement to help you without leaving her feeling overloaded or resentful. Since most girls don't make such a request—much less so politely—chances are that she'll remember and ask if you need to go when she's in the room. If she has a good memory and isn't too harried, she may even make sure you're OK just before going to lunch.

For dealing with a guy like me, something similar should work, particularly if you use that ever-effective ploy—the helpless female in need of a strong guy to rescue her from danger. We fall for that every time. Remember, it's risky for me to say or do things that get me out of work. Nurses hate that. But if you make a request, that's different. As staff, we are trained to listen carefully to patients and remember everything. And while we may seem to be the ones who're giving all the orders, a big part of our job is meeting your needs. "I need a glass of water" isn't supposed to be met with, "Get it yourself, you lazy slob."

When you talk to that guy, just be careful not to imply that you think he's weird, much less perverted. Make your shyness and fear of embarrassment the reason, and that should endear you to him. And no, that embarrassment claim doesn't mean that you turn glowing pink with the slightest skin exposure. It simply means that you don't want certain things to happen.

Remember, show you trust this guy by putting this as a request for his help. Say something like, "I'm rather shy [or easily embarrassed]. You're such a wonderful, helpful guy. Could you, whenever possible, get the nurse take care of the bedpan [or other embarrassing thing]. I'd appreciate that very much." Then throw him your biggest and best smile. If he's like me, he'd regard that as a compliment and do everything he can to help. If that nurse is about to go to lunch, he may remember to ask her to check in on you.

Most important of all, your bladder won't explode into a million pieces. That's good for all of us. Exploding bladders can be very messy. Housekeeping has to be called to clean up, and there's a ton of paperwork to be filled out.

The importance of getting staff on your side is why I'll soon be telling you how to be like a wonderful boy called Binky and become everyone's favorite patient. That'll make them eager to handle your wishes and is the golden secret to enjoying your stay. If a nurse thinks you're "an absolute sweetheart," it makes it far easier to get her to do favors for you.

My Wobbly Soapbox

I hope what I've said helps. Unfortunately, requests for favors like these are necessary because embarrassment doesn't rank very high on the 'look out for' scale at most modern hospitals. They're very medically minded. They focus on getting sick people well with drugs, surgery and therapy. In comparison to that, your blushing toes seem like nothing. But something of lesser importance isn't something of no importance. Fear and pain are of lesser importance than dying, but hospitals still take the time and trouble to deal with them. They need to learn to do the same with embarrassment.

In fact, I believe embarrassment effects patients much like pain. Both are unpleasant and something we try to avoid. If anything, we can forget something physical (meaning pain) more easily than we can forget something psychological (such as embarrassment). That's why I suspect the memory of an embarrassment is likely to linger far longer than that of a pain. That's not good.

Yes, it's true that for pain there's often a pill, while there's no pill for embarrassment. But the treatment for embarrassment—a little kindness and some staff flexibility—is more effective than that for pain. It also costs nothing and has no bad side effects. That's why I think hospitals should treat embarrassment as seriously as they do pain. Embarrassment management should be as much a part of good hospital care as pain management. There, I have said it. It's out of my system. Now I feel better. Whew!

I'd better get off my soapbox. This book is for you and not hospital administrators or staff. I must stay practical. I'm not a medical or nursing school professor or a hospital administrator. I can't change hospitals myself, but I can help you and maybe, through you, change hospitals for the better. Keep that in mind and see your time in the hospital—with all its potential for embarrassment—as a challenge and an adventure. You can make a success of it. You can make a difference!

With the Post-Op Girls and the Twins you've seen the extremes and with the Sensible Girls you've seen what's between. But even taken together the three groups don't fully represent the incredibly rich variety of girls I cared for. I'll now talk about someone who'd just been overwhelmed by the worst news imaginable. The girls we've talked about until now could make choices about how they were treated. Pala couldn't. She was totally overwhelmed.

14. OVERWHELMED PALA

I remember Pala well. She was a lovely, slender blonde of about fourteen who'd been diagnosed with leukemia two days earlier. Part of the workup for her treatment was a spinal tap, so my nurse asked me to assist a resident (doctor-in-training) in the examination room.

Curled Up Like a Baby

As always with such procedures, Pala was asked to lie on her side, curled up in a fetal position, so the resident could insert a needle into the small of her back. It's a scary procedure, not helped by the fact that she had two strange men standing over her: the resident behind to insert the needle and me, close in front, to pin her down at the waist and upper legs, so she couldn't move suddenly. There wasn't much I could do to make it better, but I did create a makeshift surgical drape out of a towel, so she'd feel less exposed.

Unfortunately for her, this resident was incompetent. Four times he poked her and four times he failed to get spinal fluid. Then he stalked off, leaving me to deal with a distraught girl. When I cleaned up, I discovered that the lumbar puncture kit he'd been using was clearly labeled for infants only. He hadn't been able to get fluid because the needle wasn't long enough.

I was furious. No matter how tired, I always thought about what I was doing, checking and rechecking everything. That's one reason I worked at the hospital for over two years, taking care of some of its most seriously ill patients, without making a single mistake serious enough to trigger an incident report. Now I had to deal with the aftermath of a dolt who couldn't get through a single day without a serious blunder. Groan!

Calm down, I told myself. You have a badly traumatized girl to care for. Think about her. I could smell urine, so I knew she'd wet herself during the procedure and wouldn't want to go back to her room smelling like that. That put me in a terrible bind. It was mid-afternoon, and this clueless resident had already put me some twenty minutes behind. Helping Pala clean up would put me even further behind. Despite their lighter work load, evening shift wouldn't be happy if I left work for them and might complain to our ill-tempered head nurse.

On the medical unit, I'd dealt with numberless little kids who'd wet themselves, so I knew there were two basic ways to change Pala. One was quick and efficient, essentially undressing and dressing her myself. She was in shock by all that had happened over the past two days and wouldn't protest. The other way would take twice as long, since I would turn around while she slowly changed and washed herself, but it would protect her feelings. She might be in a hospital, but inside she was the same fourteen-year-old girl she'd been three days earlier. If I did things the quick way, she'd feel humiliated. If I did them the gentle way, I might get yelled at.

I groaned. Why wasn't there support for treating her gently? None of the nurses would have the slightest problem if I, a guy, had dealt with Pala the quick way. Changing clothes was one of my jobs, and being an aide meant I was officially neither male nor female. Just do it, the system said.

Efficiency Above All Else

First things first. After all Pala had been through, I was worried that she might faint, so I told her to continue lying on examination table, not moving until I returned with towels and a change of clothes. That gave me a minute to think.

I knew the system stood ready to punish me for taking even a few extra minutes to deal with her kindly. Administrators value efficiency above all else, particularly above acts of kindness.

There's a sad reason for that. Unfortunately for you and I, some of those who go into nursing find that they don't like patients and escape by moving into the lower levels of nursing administration. There they discover that they don't like nurses either and make life difficult for those under them, often while pandering to their bosses. So if your nurses or their assistants seem worn out and discouraged, one of these people-haters may be behind it all. Unfortunately, you can't fire that head nurse, but you can show those who're caring for you a little kindness.

A people-hater was exactly the quandary I was in. Recently, the head nurse had called me in for a talk. A few days before, she said sternly, I'd wasted several minutes talking with a boy and his family about the hospital's closed-circuit movies-on-demand system. I should have been changing bed linen, she said.

I felt like screaming "You idiot!"—which was certainly true. I remembered that day all too well. Like Pala, the boy had just been diagnosed with leukemia. The day before, he and his family had been told that, without treatment, his leukemia was always fatal. He had been

been rushed to our hospital and admitted to the floor in the early afternoon. There the boy and his parents waited and waited and waited.

It was early afternoon of the next day when I decided to explain movies-on-demand to them in a desperate attempt to ease their anxiety. They'd been in the hospital for some twenty-fours hours, terrified about the future, and had yet to talk with one of our leukemia specialists. A resident had briefly stopped by, explained that there was an important medical conference going on, and hurried off. That was all.

Getting that boy and his family distracted by movies had incurred the wrath of a head nurse who didn't bother to investigate, so I knew I could expect little mercy if I were seen tarrying with Pala and again 'wasting time' by being kind.

A Gentler Approach

Pala was still lying down when I returned, so I helped her stand. I knew what was right. I would take the gentler, more modest approach. Anything else would be cruel to a girl who was going through hell.

Two days before she'd been told she had a cancer that could kill her. The day before she'd heard about her grim treatment options—chemotherapy drugs that might cause other cancers later in life. Today, there'd been this incompetent resident. Come what may, I would not add one drop to her already overflowing cup of misery. I could only hope that, as she thought about all that happened during the day just before falling asleep, the extra time I took now might be a tiny bright spot in an otherwise bleak day.

Yet even that decision, right as it was, has regrets. Looking back, I realize that, if I'd been a bit more clever, I might have managed a change that was both quick and gentle, perhaps with an added bit of humor for a girl whose life had suddenly become devoid of all happiness.

Instead of waiting for her to change gowns, I could have loosened the strings on the back of her wet gown, all the time stressing to her not to let it slip down, "because I embarrass easily." Then I'd stand in front of her, holding the new gown high, so I could only see her face, and saying, "Now I can only see your beautiful eyes. Let the old gown slip down—I'll pick it up later—and slip into this one." Her own fears of embarrassment would have been transformed into a joke about my own embarrassment. Rather than being overpowered by events, she'd have a chance to control them and even help me. Gosh only knows how powerless she must have felt at that moment.

Alas, I didn't think of that. I was already deviating from the system in a big way. Deviating still further, making a silly game out of a standard procedure, didn't come to me. Efficiency and humor don't mix well. Nor does creativity come easily in an environment increasingly filled with criticism. Sad.

Overwhelmed and Vulnerable

Her name, of course, wasn't really Pala. I picked it because it's one Icelanders give a girl who is small. It fits because the real girl I cared for, in her great vulnerability, stands for all those in a hospital who are overwhelmed by events and often made to do things they dislike or find embarrassing. Unable to defend herself or make her wishes clear, Pala needed a friend who wasn't under the same pressure. She needed someone who could be strong for her. That's what I was that afternoon.

Just keep in mind how special my presence was that day. When first diagnosed, children and teens with leukemia don't usually look sick, so they don't automatically trigger sympathy from hospital staff like someone in an automobile accident might. Pala looked like a teen you might see at any shopping mall. To many of my fellow workers, she would just seem a silly girl who'd wet herself during a common procedure. "Hurry up!" might be their attitude. They weren't being cruel. They simply didn't have the personal experience to understand her great hurt, and they had far too much to do. Hospital work is hard and demanding. It's easy to forget to sympathize.

But I'd had different experiences, and they shaped how I responded to Pala. I'd spent almost a year-and-a-half caring for children with leukemia who were a little younger than she was. I knew in my bones the horrors of the disease. Treatment for leukemia, then and now, works best for children at the peak age for the disease, which is about four. As a teen, Pala's chances of surviving were significantly less than for the children I'd cared for on Hem-Onc. She might have a less than 50 percent chance of being alive a year from that day. That was reason enough to brave a head nurse's wrath.

The chemotherapy she would receive in the next few days would be brutal. After that, her lovely hair would fall out and her blood counts—red, white and platelets—would plummet to dangerously low levels. She'd become so medically fragile, she could be killed by an infection that wouldn't even make you or I sick.

Even worse, for months this poor girl would receive no good news of any importance. At six months, she might be told that her cancer was still in remission, but then again she might not. Because I felt all that in my gut, because I'd lived with that reality night after night for many months, I knew she deserved every scrap of kindness I could muster. I knew she shouldn't be embarrassed or humiliated in any way. If the head nurse went ballistic—tough for her.

I hope you never face a situation like Pala's, particularly an illness that serious. But you may find yourself at a hospital with an injury or illness that leaves you feeling as overwhelmed, vulnerable, and helpless as she did that afternoon. Take hope.

Next, I'll explain how to respond to your hospitalization in a way that will attract sympathy and create a wonderful bubble of protection around you. Much as I did that afternoon with Pala, you can find hospital staff who'll go to great effort to protect you until you have the strength and resources to care for yourself. Even when you're defenseless, you don't have to be friendless.

15. MUCH-LOVED BINKY

The first time I went to Binky's bed, I saw a homemade sign at the foot saying, "I know I'm special because God don't make no junk." Whoever made the sign, his mother or a nurse, was right. He was special.

Binky was about four years old. With spindly limbs and a swollen belly, he looked like the Kermit the Frog doll that someone had left in his bed. Medically, he had Prune Belly Syndrome. Translated, that meant his belly was a mess. The name comes from the fact that, born without abdominal muscles, the belly of a baby with the syndrome can be as wrinkled as a dried prune. Binky was also missing some organs. He had only one kidney and no bladder. His diaper needed to be placed near his belly button, because that was where the urine dribbled out, one drop at a time.

Doting on Binky

Yet despite all the added work Binky created for staff, he was an absolute joy to care for. Just coming up to his bed would make me feel better. I still remember one day when the order came to remove the NG (nasogastric, meaning nose-to-stomach) tube we'd been using to feed him formula. The tube itself is soft and doesn't hurt when in place.

But going down and coming up, it creates a choking sensation as the tip passes through the lower throat. I was trying to be careful with that when he expressed concern for me. In spite of all he was going through, he was more worried about my feelings than his own. That was Binky, a most incredible kid.

As you might expect, the nursing staff doted on this wonderful little guy and, given the severity of his sickness, quite a few staff throughout the hospital got to know him. His dying was a long, downward spiral. His one kidney began to fail, dialysis was impossible for anyone as frail as he, and every effort to adjust his diet came to naught. The night he died, one of the evening aides—on her own initiative and on her on time—stayed to be with him, holding his hand until his family arrived.

After his death, his family, knowing how special he was to the staff, held a memorial service just for us. They knew our shifts and picked the best possible time, which was in early afternoon. But that only meant that attending was equally difficult for everyone. For those on nights like me it meant getting up at what our bodies thought was three a.m. For those on days, it meant finding someone willing to come in early to cover for them. For those on evenings, it meant finding someone on days who'd stay over until they could get to work. The result was a lot of people making a special effort to honor one amazing little boy. For our other children, the most nursing staff I saw attend a funeral was about six. No less that twenty-four nurses and aides came to honor little Binky's short but impressive life.

Why so Special?

Why were so many people willing to give something extra to care for Binky while he was alive and to make a special effort to honor him after he was dead? Sick and frail, little Binky had nothing of material value to give us. It was the little things he did all the time, particularly the appreciation he showed for what we did for him. When I did something, he'd thank me, even when he was so weak, he could barely gasp out the words. You cared about him because he cared about you.

Why did that create such strong bonds? In part, it was because, strange as it sounds, expressing gratitude and showing concern for caregivers are rare in hospitals. Does that mean our patients didn't appreciate what we were doing? Not at all. I had a number of kids who liked me. I remember a little girl from Hem-Onc whose mother brought her by to see me on the teen unit after my transfer. As soon as the girl saw me, she threw herself out of her mother's arms and into mine. She was delighted to see the guy who'd sung her to sleep, night after night, with those terrible, off-key renditions of "You are my sunshine."

No, the problem wasn't a lack of appreciation. The appreciation was there. It was just that these kids, from babies to teens, often faced problems so overwhelming it was difficult for them to take their eyes off their fears and suffering. We were strong, we were healthy, and we seemed so emotionally together. What could they give us? What need did we have for anything they might do? And yet we did, as the amazing response to Binky reveals. We needed to see and hear their thanks and appreciation.

Care for Those Caring for You

That's the essence of the magic tip I'm offering you. When you're in a hospital and feeling overwhelmed, take a moment to say something kind to those caring for you. Thank them even for little things. If a nurse reaches over and adjusts your pillow, show your appreciation. If you're so sick, you can barely gasp out the words, the nurse will be even more impressed. If those caring for you seemed stressed out—as they usually are—say something like, "I can tell you're busy today. Thanks for helping me."

Remember, you're stuck in that bed with nothing else to do. You might as well be kind and thoughtful. It certainly beats being crabby and critical. Look for ways to compliment staff. If the hospital allows a nurse to dress distinctively, find something to praise about her outfit. When I worked with little kids, I clipped a little Kola bear to my stethoscope to make it more friendly. If you see something like that, mention it. Take the time to see them as people. Learn their names and something about them. Remember their days off and mention missing them when they come back. If a nurse said something about going for a hike, ask her how it went. She's caring for you. Show you care about her.

Show Humor

Don't forget humor, which can work wonders in tense situations. Look online for stories about how President Ronald Reagan responded after almost being killed by an assassin. As a patient, he impressed everyone who came in contact with him. When he first arrived at the Georgetown Hospital ER, he was bleeding so badly internally that he drifted in and out of consciousness. Half his blood had to be replaced by transfusions. And yet one time when he briefly regained consciousness, he noticed a nurse was holding his hand and joked with her, "Does Nancy [his wife] know about us?"

Shortly after that, he was taken into surgery to remove a bullet that had stopped an mere inch from his heart. His doctors were worried and tense. None wanted to be known as the one whose mistake killed a President. To ease their tension, Reagan quipped that he hoped they all were Republicans, to which the head surgeon replied something like, "Today, Mr. President, we're all Republicans." With Reagan, everyone who cared for him felt his interest in them. During the weeks he spent in the hospital recovering, he spent his nights joking with his nurses. It's easy to see why they adored a patient who gave them so much attention.

You can do the same. As a teen girl, you can be incredibly infuriating or wonderfully charming. (Just ask your mother.) The choice is yours, so pick the latter. Show your appreciation and demonstrate an interest in those caring for you. Take difficult situations with humor, remembering that it's always safe to make jokes about yourself. If something unpleasant happens, try laughing about it rather than throwing a snit or sulking. A good sense of humor is always appealing.

Care for Other Patients

Finally, don't forget to care for the patients around you. Your nurses will notice and appreciate that too. At one point, one of our rooms had so many girls with 'head' issues, my nurse referred to it as a "psychiatric ward." Yet a new girl transformed everything with her interest in the other girls. Even more surprising, she was someone you might think would have had the worst problems of all.

Cheryl was about fifteen, with warm and caring blue eyes. She'd been so badly abused as a baby, one nurse told me that she still had scars on her buttocks from where cigarettes had been snuffed out. Even worse, one of her legs had been so badly broken, it was several inches shorter than the other, causing her to walk with a limp. She only escaped those horrors because a kind and loving couple adopted her.

That short leg brought her into our care. We had a surgery just for her. On the first visit, our surgeons would stop the growth in her longer leg. Then a year or so later, when the shorter leg reached that same length, they'd stop the growth in it. Cheryl would end up a little shorter, but she'd have two legs the same length and a normal walk. That's good.

I still have a picture of her in a wheelchair made when I took her and her mother down to go home. I remember telling myself that, if I'd been a boy of sixteen, she'd have been getting my attention. She was that special. You could do worse than be like her.

Someone Else in Need

You might also read books for inspiration. If you like romances, particularly the true-life ones, you might read *A Severe Mercy* by Sheldon Vanauken. The book is about his much-loved wife, Davy. At one point in her illness, it became clear that she would die so, as he put it, she began to say, "farewell to the wind and sky, watching it all go and fade away, die—and thanking God. And yet she was human, heartbreakingly human, and she did not want to die." He continues:

> She obediently did everything the doctors and the nurses told her to do: everything except to stay in her bed when someone else was in need. Over and over again, she was discovered out of bed in the night, sitting beside some other patient who was suffering, soothing her, holding her hand, praying for her.... Later I would get dozens of letters, some almost illiterate, from people who had been in the hospital with her, saying that she had helped and sustained them. One said she was like an angel of God.
>
> The nurses loved her and the hospital servants, too. She enlisted my help to make a grand medal, "for faithful service" for one of the black maids, who wore it proudly. Many of the nurses were praying for her.... It is simply true, without exaggeration, to say that she was a tower of strength to everyone.... Love shone forth from her, and love not only begets love, it transmits strength.

Always remember something important about hospitals. Many of those who enter medicine and nursing are caring people. They wouldn't have chosen the work if they weren't. But the sheer burden of it all, emotionally and physically, often overcomes them. On top of that, hospitals are filled to the brim with suffering and tragedy. The staff, overwhelmed by their work and surrounded by so much pain, often feel they must wall out that sadness out to cope. Treating them as special breaks down those walls. Being as funny as you can manage and showing concern for other patients also helps. You become special. They'll notice you, care for you, and protect you in the tough times.

That's my magic tip. It's incredibly simple. Like Binky, be a joy to those caring for you. Become their favorite patient and they will look out for you.

Next, we'll look at a girl who was in a situation much like Pala's, but in much worse shape emotionally. Broken Tina was what I didn't want Pala to become. Not ever.

16. Broken Tina

I was still on the medical unit, and it was about five a.m. Someone was moving around behind Tina's drawn curtains. When I went to check, I found that her mother had just finished changing the sheets. Tina had wet herself in her sleep. I felt rotten. No one likes to do that, particularly not a twelve-year-old girl.

As always when something went askew, I asked myself what I could have done to prevent it. Tina had leukemia and was staying with us overnight before being transferred to the teen unit to begin a second round of chemotherapy. Since she'd yet to start treatment, her doctor had written a Q8 order for vital signs. That meant I was to check her at the start of the shift and then leave her alone to sleep through the night, which is what I'd done. We didn't get too many Q8s on the medical unit. A child sick enough to be hospitalized generally needed to be checked every four hours (Q4). Kids sicker than that were almost always sent to the ICU, where Q2 was the norm.

Tina's Haste

As first, I blamed myself for not making clear to Tina that, if she needed a bedpan, I was as willing to get the nurse as to do it myself. She'd probably seen only me, I thought, and concluded she had a guy for a nurse. Later in the night, when she woke up needing to go, she'd decided, "No, I don't want a guy doing this," and gone back to sleep. Then in her sleep she'd wet herself. That was plausible and had the advantage of offering a fix for what had gone wrong—always make clear to these older girls that they had a woman nurse as an option.

The problem was that it didn't fit with Tina's earlier, way-outside-the-norm behavior. When I'd come up to her bed just before midnight for that Q8 check, she'd asked for a bedpan, which I pulled from under the bed and slid underneath her. Most patients, guys or girls, would then wait for me to do something. After Maria, I'd have slipped down her undies beneath her gown and helped her sit up. Tina didn't wait. Despite having only met me seconds earlier, she sat up, shoved down her sheet, pulled her gown above her waist, and slipped down her panties. Not the usual girlish behavior.

Something similar happened at five a.m. As I talked with her mother, Tina was sitting up in bed and listening to the two of us, while wearing little more than what her mother would have called a 'trainer bra.'

I don't pretend to understand teen girls, much less those just entering puberty, but it seemed odd at the time that she made no effort to turn away or at least cover herself. And if she didn't embarrass that easily, my theory about why she'd wet herself fell apart. That left me with no reason for what went wrong and no fix for this sort of bedwetting. That bothered me. A problem left unfixed could happen again.

Breaking Tina

While writing this book, I reexamined that night, and think I now understand what happened. Fretting about her upcoming chemotherapy, Tina slept poorly her last few nights at home. That's understandable. She'd gone through it before and knew how awful it is. In the hospital, her waiting now over, she'd fallen into an exhausted sleep and hadn't awakened when she should. That happened often enough, mothers often asked us to wake their kids in the night to see if they needed to go.

That leaves for explanation only Tina's seeming eagerness to expose herself in front of me, a total stranger. Later, I'll describe the embarrassment I saw in Ginny's eyes when I inadvertently saw her topless. What I saw in Tina's eyes that night wasn't embarrassment. It more like a deep sense of defeat, sadness, and the like coupled with a grim determination to live. Before her leukemia, I'm sure she'd been like most other girls her young age, meaning shy about that sort of thing. But her illness had altered her, breaking her spirit in some terrible way. That, I now believe, was our crime.

Tina's brokenness is why I decided to closely follow the story about Pala with this one about Tina, even though the latter happened some months earlier. The two girls are so closely linked as to be almost inseparable. Both had leukemia and both were so traumatized by their treatment that they wet themselves—Tina the day before her chemotherapy and Pala during her spinal tap. These were girls under enormous pressure. Even more important, both faced a serious possibility of dying in mere months. As a result, both felt unable to resist how they were treated by a system that offered them a chance at life. That's the essence of the problem as I see it.

Tina, battling for her life, was what I instinctively feared Pala might become. Recall what I chose not to do with Pala. To protect her, I refused to take off her gown and pull down her panties to save myself a little time, even though that was standard hospital practice and delay might get me a rebuke. Now recall what Tina did. In front of me, she flipped up her gown and pulled down her panties merely to save a few seconds over waiting for me. I'd refused to give Pala the standard treatment. Tina was re-enacting that same standard treatment in front of me. To understand why Tina acted that way, it helps to grasp what she and other girls like her endure in the weeks after their leukemia or some other serious illness is diagnosed.

After a Deadly Diagnosis

The first circumstance that comes after a deadly diagnosis is a sense of being completely and utterly overwhelmed. That's what Pala was experiencing that afternoon. So much had happened, all of it terrible, that her ability to cope had simply shut down. That's why I knew she wouldn't resist if I changed her clothes the quick way. That's also why I chose the gentle way rather than offer her a choice like I might with some girls, given my need to hurry. Pala was in no condition to choose, so I had to be her friend and do what was best for her.

Picture yourself in a similar situation, and you'll realize just how hard it would have been for her to assert herself. She was in utter, complete shock. Her experience is why I stress the need to make friends among the staff as soon as you arrive at a hospital. You need someone experienced and strong looking out for you—someone who will do for you what you can't do for yourself.

The second circumstance flows inexorably from the first. Told that you have an illness that can kill you, you cling desperately to whatever offers hope. Think of a drowning person grabbing at anything that floats. That's what I sensed, more than anything else, about Tina that night. She was desperately afraid of dying, so desperate she was willing to do anything to live. You and I might feel exactly the same.

That willingness is good to the extent that it means that patients endure all the horrors of treatment. It's certainly not true that the treatment for leukemia is worse than the disease itself. Left untreated, dying with leukemia is often accompanied by a stokes and seizures, which are terrible ways to die. I saw that one night with a young boy. But it's also true that for many months after someone is diagnosed, the treatment will *feel* much worse than the disease had been. That desperation to live helps girls such as Tina endure all that misery.

Unfortunately, those life-saving treatments come with a third circumstance—additional hospital-imposed baggage that has nothing to do with curing leukemia or any other disease. Those are the hospital policies, procedures, and practices about patient care, particularly those that some patients find embarrassing or that violate their sense of self.

Those who created those practices are not evil or perverse. I certainly wasn't before Maria. We are just blind and clueless to their potential results and obsessed with being quick at getting our work done.

Staff Are Not Male or Female

Yes, those practices exist to make work in the hospital flow smoothly and efficiently. The most glaring of them is the worst, the one I call 'staff are not male or female.' It simplified our work enormously. Staff could be assigned with no regard to a patient's sex or feelings about that. If something needed to be done, anyone could do it, even if I was a thirty-ish guy and she was a twelve-year-old girl just passing through puberty. Simple, direct, and efficient—just what administrators like, and what a nursing staff with a heavy workload feel they must do. That's the key reason why some may resist the changes I suggest here.

With the children we cared for on Hem-Onc, that mattered little. To our young patients, the nurse and I weren't female and male. We were like their mommy and daddy, and that's how they responded. In fact, one of the first occasions when I realized that wasn't always true came one unhappy night when I floated to the teen unit.

There, one of my patients was Julie, a brown-haired girl of about seventeen who was being treated for leukemia. Her IV was running fast, as it typically did with someone getting chemotherapy, and someone on staff had blundered, putting a child-sized bedpan in her room. Her mother, not knowing any better, had used it. When the mother saw it was almost overflowing, she panicked and called me. I did my best to slip it out from under Julie without spilling, moving slowly and carefully. I even worked from the side, where all I could see were her hips, hoping to avoid embarrassing her. Unfortunately, despite my efforts to be kind, I failed completely and utterly. Throughout the long, clumsy process, Julie was sobbing from embarrassment, leaving me feeling like a jerk. The only way I could make amends was to get an adult-sized bedpan from supply and give it to the mom, so the problem wouldn't happen again.

Imagine Yourself

Now imagine yourself in either Julie's situation or that of Tina. You have a serious illness, one that can kill you, and one that requires a long and exhausting hospitalization. Around the clock, staff come into your room, some men and some women. If you need something, however personal and private, you're expected to accept assistance from whoever is available, even if that leaves you feeling exposed and violated. That's why Julie endured my help despite her obvious distress. It's also why that night it never occurred to me to get the nurse to deal with that overfilled bedpan. Julie and I were in a situation we both hated but that seemed unavoidable. At the time, I was as trapped in that culture she was.

The same was true of Tina when she was being treated on that same teen unit, perhaps even in that same room. Her bladder filled around the clock from her fast IV. When that happened, she'd flip on the call light, not knowing if a man or woman would come. Whichever it was, the procedure was always the same—pull down her sheets, flip up her gown, and slip down her panties. Over and over again. That's why she'd done just that when I'd come to her bed. She'd become as she'd been treated.

Embarrassment as Violation

I don't know what happened to either Tina or Julia. Both were my patients for just one night. But looking back, I can see what that sort of experience did to an innocent, twelve-year-old Tina, who was wrestling with all the changes that were happening to her body at puberty. It's what evil men do to young women when they want to force them into prostitution. They violate them time and again until they lose any will to resist. However Tina might have felt in her heart of hearts, after all those bedpans, she was now compliant. Fearful of dying, she did what she thought she had to do—even with complete strangers like me.

If the word "violated" seems too much, substitute "embarrassed." It doesn't matter. Tina had been embarrassed so many times by how we as staff treated her, that her will had been broken. Even the fact that I'd have done things differently if she'd waited but a few seconds made no difference. I never got a chance. She preempted anything I might do. In a sense, perhaps undressing herself in front of me was one last, desperate effort to preserve a shred of her dignity. She was doing it herself, so it couldn't be wrong. Sad, very sad.

Will this happen to you? I most certainly hope not, and this book was written to make absolutely sure it doesn't. I do think that Tina was the exception rather than the rule. I believe she was strongly affected because she was so young and passing through a special time in her life. As a fully grown woman, it might have been different. I once had a mother in her thirties tell me that, after having three kids in a hospital, she'd given up on feminine modesty. Age may be a factor in what happens.

But that doesn't mean that what happened to her couldn't happen to you or to someone you know. That's why, at the beginning of this book, I pointed out that being forewarned is forearmed. Knowing what might happen to you or a friend should allow you to take steps to keep it from happening. No matter what sickness you face, don't let your spirit get broken. Don't let any fear of death overwhelm your sense of yourself. Be yourself whatever comes.

So yes, Tina was an exception—one with horrible results. Much more common, from what I recall as I look back, was the reaction of Ginny, the girl we'll discuss next. She also offers the key to understanding why such things happen in hospitals dedicated to healing.

17. FRIGHTENED GINNY

It was mid-afternoon on the teen unit, and I was working with a girl in the far corner of a girls room, when a nurse across the room said something to me to get my attention. When I turned around, I saw that she was with a frightened, dark-haired sixteen-year-old girl whose gown lay crumpled around her waist.

I quickly turned away. "Why did you do that?," I thought to myself. "Ginny has lost half of her left arm to bone cancer. She has that central line to get chemotherapy, so her cancer doesn't spread and kill her. She has enough troubles. She doesn't need me looking at her." I was angry and took care not to turn around or leave my patient until the gown was back up and the nurse had left.

What was that central line? It's like an IV in that it's used to put fluids and medicines into a patient. But it's different in an important way. Instead of using a metal needle that typically goes into an arm vein, it uses a flexible Silastic (rubbery) tube running into a much larger vein close to the heart. A central line is wonderful for patients with a serious illness. Put in by a surgeon, it will last for months, preventing poke after poke. It can also be used to draw blood, preventing yet more pokes.

In our hospital, patients who needed lengthy treatments typically had central lines. We helped pioneer the technique, and the inventor of one of the most common central lines was one of our physicians. In most cases, including Ginny's, the central line went into their upper chest just below the right shoulder blade. Since there's a possibility of an infection, the opening in the skin had to be cleaned regularly. That was often done by specially trained nurses like the one here. I liked those nurses. They were talented and did their job well. But they were still women, with all that meant for girls, as we will see.

A Common Practice

Unfortunately, what that nurse did that afternoon is all too common in hospitals. Becoming blasé about patient nudity is a reasonable response to being surrounded by so much of it. The problem is that, while it may help staff to do their jobs more efficiently, it's not pleasant for patients, particularly not for many teen girls like you. Years of hospital experience had made that thirty-some nurse into someone who'd actually draw a guy's attention to a topless sixteen-year-old girl. But that girl did not have the benefits of her nurse's long hospital experience and never would. For her, it was humiliating. Before I turned away, I could see the fear in her eyes.

Ginny's responses—obvious fright and yet doing nothing—were so typical, you might consider them the normal ones. If you're wondering how you might react in the situations I've been describing in this book, hers is the most likely. She could see I was busily working across the room, and yet she had done nothing in advance to cover herself up or to get this nurse to keep her covered. Even when I'd turned around, she hadn't tried to cover herself, unlike what most girls her age would have done in any place other than at a hospital.

I can't explain why so many girls acted so differently in a hospital than on the outside. If something medical is happening that required exposure you don't like, gritting your teeth and enduring it makes sense. But when the exposure serves no medical purpose, when it is little more than the whim of a nurse or a gown flopping the wrong way, enduring had no reason. In those cases, covering up made more sense. And yet, embarrassed as they were, these girls—the majority of them in fact— seemed afraid to do something to cover up. As a guy, that seemed crazy.

Worse still was what might have happened that day. The nurse was inviting me into a conversation, one that would have given me an opportunity to continue to look on and even to come over and ask questions about the infection control procedures she was applying. If I'd done that, my curiosity would have been as phony as a three-dollar bill. I'd helped nurses do that same procedure on small children in Hem-Onc. I knew almost enough to do it myself. That faked attention, more than anything else, was what Ginny feared. This nurse wasn't protecting her modesty. Instead, she was inviting me to violate it. No, that nurse wasn't being deliberately cruel. I don't even think she was doing it consciously. For some reason, this nurse—and many like her—seemed blind to any embarrassment the girls in her care might feel. Soon, I'll talk more about why.

A Nurse's Perspective

Now ponder that girl's situation from the nurse's perspective. The nurse had seen me across the room when she arrived, so why was the robe around the girl's waist? That didn't have to be. The central line entered her chest just under her shoulder blades. All that nurse needed to do was loosen the gown a bit or perhaps have the girl hold it up with her good right arm. All that exposure wasn't necessary. And why had she drawn my attention? She didn't have to do that. If she wanted a conversation, she could have talked with the girl.

Even more telling was a question that haunted me during most of my time at the hospital. Why was it almost always the women on staff (both nurses and medical residents) who were creating these embarrassing situations for girls? What was going on? Wasn't there any loyalty among women? Where was their sympathetic modesty? They wouldn't like what was happening if it involved them. Why were they imposing it on these girls?

As the lone guy on the teen unit, I wrestled constantly with the guy-see-girl issues that this nurse was ignoring. I knew that just by being present, I could embarrass a girl who already had more than enough pain to bear. I didn't want to be a jerk, yet I was regularly put in those situations by women on staff. A few would ask a girl's permission before doing something with me around, but most didn't.

Assertive Nina

Of course, not all girls reacted passively. Some could defend themselves with impressive determination. A little after midnight, while I was still working on the medical unit, I got a call to pick up Nina, a girl of about sixteen who was in the emergency room suffering from severe sunburn. Although I didn't notice it at the time, as I now recall the overflow of teens to the medical unit was always girls. Maybe they sent guys to the surgical unit one floor up. That'd keep the two sexes from accidentally mixing in the same multi-bed room. The hospital's casualness about undress never applied to teen boy and girl mixing. That they'd never permit.

When I arrived at the ER, I discovered that Nina was still in the exam room with a resident who was about to apply a steroid salve to her sun-burned and soon-to-be-bare chest. The resident—yes, as usual, a woman and one I knew well—didn't seem to have any problem with my staying, but I politely excused myself and waited outside.

Arriving back at the medical unit, Nina and I went through the admission procedure, which included weighing, and that created a problem. Nina had her own jeans on but had yet to acquire a gown. The thick cotton blanket she was carefully using to cover herself was heavy enough to throw her weight off. Thinking that the fact that I'd left the exam room might have convinced her to trust me, I tried to get her to simply face away and put aside the blanket. Nothing doing, she said. So I guessed at a weight for the blanket and subtracted that from what the scale said. Given that her problem was sunburn, her weight wasn't that critical. I didn't offer to get her a gown, since she'd have probably said no again, but the next time I was in the room, I noticed that she'd gotten the nurse to get her one. This sixteen-year-old definitely didn't buy the idea that hospital staff weren't male or female. I was a guy and that was that. Good for her.

Yes, Nina was a bit more prickly and defensive than she needed to be that night. I wasn't up to any guy tricks. But I felt far more comfortable caring for her than for sad and broken little Tina, who'd been assigned to a bed across that same room on a different night. None of my blundering guyness was going to hurt the pretty, you're-not-going-to-see-me-undressed Nina. She had her guard up. In contrast, young Tina's spirit had been so broken, it was difficult for me not to hurt her, however hard I might try. Nina had probably never been hospitalized before that night, but she'd adapted quickly. In contrast, all Tina's girlish defenses had crushed by the hospital, with its dreadfully standardized unisex procedures.

No, the goal of this book isn't to make you exactly like Nina, although she could serve as a passable role model. It's to help you learn to behave just as firmly as she did, but with a confidence and politeness that'll win you friends among the staff. Being liked while being firm should be your goal. That will win you the respect and kind treatment you want.

Next, I'll explain why hospital staff act as they do about patient undress, especially the guys around girls sort. Understanding that should help you take charge of your care and may even allow you to teach your nurses something they need to learn. In fact, you might want to loan a copy of this book to one of your nurses and say, as politely as you can, "You might like to read this. It's really helped me."

18. NEEDY LENNY AND JENNIE

Perhaps the best way to understand why many of the nurses I worked with seemed indifferent to undress in teen girls is—I'm ashamed to admit—to realize that I had an identical attitude toward our teen boys. Their undress and even nudity bothered me not a whit, even in the presence of nurses who (in my case) were always women. I was precisely like the nurses whose behavior irritated me. They and I were mirror images, although I did not recognize that at the time.

That's illustrated by two similar situations, one with a boy and one with a girl, with both needing my help and both involving a bath and physical therapy. Looking back, it's obvious that, when it came to embarrassment, I was insensitive to the point of indifference with the guy and most cautious toward the girl.

Helping Lenny

Lenny was about seventeen and, although I've forget the reason, he'd had a head injury so severe, he spent a week or more in the ICU before coming to us. He didn't talk or even gesture, but was obviously aware of his surroundings, sitting up and looking at me when I spoke to him.

Over the next few days, he improved rapidly, often seeming more capable at the end of my shift than at the start. I could see he needed to get into therapy, but no one seemed to be noticing his improvements but me. It was a classic case of an easy patient being ignored. Normally, I would have worked within the system, nudging here and hinting there, but there wasn't time for that. I decided a bold move was needed. I would show everyone just how well he was doing. Then he would get the attention he deserved.

Suspecting my nurse wouldn't go along, I waited until she went to lunch. Then I filled a bathtub with warm water, slowly walked Lenny to it, and helped him in. I thought he'd be delighted by a real bath after all the sponge baths, and I was right. He loved it, turning first in one direction and then another, always being careful to keep his head out of the water. Then to my great delight, the boy's physician arrived, saw what was happening, and promised to move quickly. He was as good as his word. Lenny was transferred to the rehab unit that very afternoon.

Ah, but here comes the fun part. Lenny was enjoying his bath so much, I left him there. A few minutes later my nurse came back from lunch, noticed he was missing, and asked me where he was. Semi-comatose people, she rightly assumed, don't slip off to the cafeteria for a cup of coffee. As casually as I could, I said, "Oh, he's taking a bath." From the look she gave me, you'd have thought I'd decided to drown the guy to free up a bed. I had to show him bathing happily in the tub, before she'd believe he was OK. Notice how casual I was about showing a nurse a teen boy totally unclothed. That's me acting very medical and most professional. That's me treating a teen boy much like—as I often complained to myself—my nurses did with teen girls. I was no different. I was they. I had met the enemy, and he was me.

Helping Jenny

Contrast that with a similar situation that happened at change of shift one morning when the nurse I was working with casually asked me to help a girl named Jennie with a warm bath. For her, that was no big deal. I was staff and that was what staff did. But I immediately thought, "Yeah, but what about Jennie? How will she feel about this? I'm a guy."

Unfortunately, there were no alternatives. Report time meant everyone, both nurses and assistants, were busy with things they had to do. It was me or no one. Delay was also impossible. The bath had to be before the girl left for physical therapy in a few minutes. Jennie was my patient and thus my responsibility. It was that simple.

Compounding my dilemma, I knew the terrible circumstances that called for this bath. Jennie had been one of my patients when she'd first been diagnosed with juvenile arthritis a few months before. At that time, I couldn't even detect her problem. It took a specialist to do that. Now her stiff movements were obvious even to my untrained eyes. She was a pretty girl with a trim, athletic figure, just the sort you could imagine becoming a cheerleader or the captain of a girl's soccer team.

But that would never be. Juvenile arthritis is one of the cruelest of diseases. We could actually cure leukemia, but there is no cure for juvenile arthritis. Even the best of treatment still meant she'd be severely disabled for the rest of her life. The thought of her in a few years— her frame distorted by arthritis and her steps halting and painful—was heartbreaking. Anything that would help her was worth doing.

Getting help was why Jennie was in for therapy. I'd talked with therapists who worked with patients like her. They told me how critical it was to get these kids to brave their pain, to do their exercises, and to keep up their mobility. Fear of pain kept them from doing what they needed to do, which reduced their mobility and increased their pain, which then further decreased their mobility in a terrible downward spiral. She was in for just a few days. Letting her have a warm soak just before her therapy would make big difference.

And no, there was no modesty workaround like there was with linen changes or bedpans. Jennie could not undress herself. She was so stiff, I'd have to help her with everything. I did draw one line though. My nurse was afraid she'd try to get out of the tub on her own and fall. I pled busyness as an excuse to leave her alone, since I knew my real reason would carry little weight. Getting her into and out of the tub was necessary. I was fine with that. Staying around watching—or rather not watching—her bathe was not. I was sure she'd rather be alone for that. Instead, I stressed to Jennie the importance of using the call light to get me when she needed to get out. That'd also be a good test to see if she was comfortable with our arrangement.

In the end, all went well. I did what I could to reassure her. I moved quickly. I looked her in the eyes as much as possible, and I talked to her. She was in for several days of therapy, so I promised myself that if I sensed any uneasiness from her, I'd come up with some alternative for those other days. That wasn't necessary.

The Contrast

Notice the great contrast between my casualness about showing my nurse the boy Lenny in the bath and my nurse's casualness about my getting the girl Jennie into a bath. She and I were thinking and acting alike, with only the sex of the patients changed.

Next, we'll look at why medical and nursing training creates those attitudes. For now, keep in mind that this matters to you because it's a part of the system that determines how you'll be treated in a hospital—that is if you don't do something to change things. In the end, it's all up to you. I can tell you what to do, but you must do it.

19. BRAVE AMY

Patients in comas require lots of care. That's why I was delighted when Amy, a nursing student, was brave enough to pick a fourteen-year-old boy in a long-term coma as her patient for the day. Almost without exception, female nursing students took girls as their patients. That's understandable. Our high school boys were only a little younger than guys they might be dating. But I was less than happy that most of these nursing students also avoided difficult patients. "I have almost a dozen teens to care for," I would grumble to myself, "while they only need to care for one. Couldn't they at least pick my most time-consuming patient?" This nurse-to-be, bless her dear heart, was doing just that.

A Boy in a Coma

Amy's patient for the day, Jeff, had been in a coma for some three months following a dirt bike accident on an Oregon sand dune. The family said that once or twice he'd spoken a few words, but, if so, he was seriously 'locked in,' rarely able to communicate with others. From time to time he would get upset, with his heart rate, breathing and blood pressure skyrocketing. He was a difficult patient, so I was glad to have her take him on.

That day he became even more difficult for brave Amy. Jeff was being fed through a NG tube with a milk-like formula, so his stool was enormous, soft and messy. The only good news was that it didn't smell.

We were a teaching hospital, so I knew exactly what I was expected to do—teach. I helped, but I made sure that unfortunate nurse-to-be did the diaper change herself. That's an unavoidable part of being a nurse, I told myself, something she needs to learn. I wasn't being mean. What I was making her do, she'd have to do as a nurse.

Why did I make Amy do something that was much harder for her than me? Because medical training includes a large, and for the most part necessary, dose of desensitization. Things that ordinary people avoid—such as open wounds, blood, bodily excretions, and even pain—are things that doctors, nurses and other medical staff must learn to deal with calmly and dispassionately. If you're in a car accident and are rushed to a hospital bleeding badly, you don't want the ER physician turning pale, muttering "Oh no, blood," and collapsing on the floor.

Hospital staff are also taught to block out normal emotional responses to nudity. I've already mentioned that it was the female nurses and residents with whom I worked who seemed the most willing to undress a teen girl when I was around. "Why don't women look out for one another better?" I'd ask myself. "They'd certainly be embarrassed if they were put in this situation. Don't they feel any sympathy for these girls? These girls clearly don't like this."

Desensitization Training

Desensitization is why. It's also, alas, why I behaved in the same callous fashion when the patient was a boy. That's because the same-sex side of desensitization is easy. For most of us, same-sex nudity is no big deal. We're not hormonally programmed to react to it, and we go through high school showering with our own sex. If we add that pre-existing tilt to the sort of desensitization that those in medicine and nursing are taught, we can see why hospital staff so easily brush aside their sympathetic modesty when the person is someone of their our own sex. In fact, as staff we seemed proud that we were 'professional' enough to not be concerned about such things. It's an easy virtue to acquire.

The difficult part of desensitization comes when the exposure involves someone of the opposite sex. There our hormones and youthful experiences work against us. There, I'm afraid all this well-intentioned indoctrination doesn't work quite as well as everyone pretends. We try, but as hospital staff our humanness still shapes how we act, consciously or unconsciously, as well as for good or ill. That's why my own frustrations with those casual, trusting Post-Op Girls weren't all that different from how the nurses I worked with responded to similar situations involving teen boys.

Nurses and Guys

Take, for example, my wanting to have a woman aide help me with bed linen changes for those Post-Op Girls. That's like a nurse who wanted my help placing a urine catheter in a boy of about 18 who was paralyzed from the waist down. I went with her, knowing ahead of time that there wasn't anything in the procedure that needed my help. She simply wanted me around to make her feel more comfortable about what she was doing, and I don't fault her for that. I was there to give her emotional and moral support.

Another occasion was like my avoiding placing a bedpan under that late-afternoon Post-Op Girl. In this situation, the patient was a strong and muscular black guy in his early twenties in a sickle cell crisis so severe, the large doses of pain-killers he was getting had rendered him unconscious. For some reason, he didn't have a gown or underpants on so, as he thrashed about in his pain, he kicked away the sheet that was his only covering. For me, that was no big deal. When I'd check in on him, I'd simply replace the sheet and move on.

Alas, that afternoon I was as dense as a tree stump. Unfairly, I got frustrated with my nurse for not doing her job. "He's getting a huge dose of morphine," I told myself. "She should be checking on him more often." Yeah, like she wanted to be all alone behind a curtain looking at an unconscious guy almost her age with absolutely nothing on. Even a moment's reflection would have told me that, if the roles had been reversed, I'd have been as evasive as she was. I should have shown her sympathy and support. We were a team, and I wasn't carrying my share of the load. I could have easily put adult diaper on the guy. It'd have meant nothing to me, but would have made her job far easier.

Unfortunately, the prevailing culture at our hospital—and probably most modern hospitals—assumes that sensitivity problem has been trained away. To admit that opposite-sex nudity unsettles, much less embarrasses you, is like admitting that you get queasy at the sight of blood. It seems unprofessional and perhaps even an admission of incompetence.

Squelching Conversations

That's not all. That hospital culture also squelches conversation between staff. That's why the nurse I was working with that day couldn't tell me, "Hey, could you put something on this guy? Naked like that, he embarrasses me." Absence those words from her, I didn't realize that what wasn't a problem for me was a huge problem for her. Her silence toward me was precisely like my silence toward nurses about my frustrations with those lovable but ill-clad Post-Op Girls. I needed help and knew it, but I couldn't ask. I only got help with their linen changes because one of my fellow assistants, a dear woman, seemed to sense my discomfort with those changes—probably because I was delaying doing them—and volunteered to help.

The oddest fact was that those same nurses and I didn't have any trouble talking about the most intimate subjects. I've had conversations with nurses on almost every topic imaginable. A labor and delivery nurse I once dated loved to talk about delivering babies, tubal ligations, and C-Sections. A pretty single nurse on Hem-Onc told me, in graphic detail, how when she was twelve, doctors fixed her too-small urethea (the tube from the bladder to the outside). When I discovered that a nine-year-old girl I'd helped to the toilet just had her period, I had no problem telling her nurse. Nurses are not inhibited in the slightest.

Embarrassment Taboos

That lack of inhibition is not surprising. Frank discussions about sex and anatomy aren't the problems they were a century and more ago.

Now it's the opposite extreme that has become an unspeakable taboo. Embarrassment, exposure, and modesty aren't discussed—especially not in hospitals. We've become the mirror image of those much-mocked nineteenth-century Victorians. What they wouldn't talk about, sex and anatomy, we talk about constantly. What they talked about all the time, modesty and embarrassment, we're afraid to mention.

Unbelievable as it may sound, during my some twenty-six months at the hospital, I can't recall a single staff conversation about a patient's embarrassment or feelings of modesty. We could talk about dying. We could talk about pain. We could talk about gruesome diseases and intrusive procedures. We did that all the time. What we couldn't talk about was one of the most normal and natural of human feelings. Looking back, it seems strange.

Worse still, our silence hurt our most vulnerable patients, particularly the younger and more vulnerable teens such as Min, Pala, and Tina. Each of those girls had enough trouble in her life. They didn't need our blundering, yank-off-their-sheets, pull-down-their-undies techniques. And to be fair, the guys, surrounded by an almost all female staff, didn't need my indifference to their nudity any more than the girls needed that of our female nurses and residents. This bizarre embarrassment about embarrassment kept us from working together. Our reticence hurt our patients, particularly the younger and more vulnerable ones.

Fortunately, understanding why a problem exists can go a long way toward dealing with it. Keep these training-induced fears in mind when you're in the hospital and show a little understanding for those caring for you. We're not as cruel, indifferent, or even perverted as we may seem at times. We're often just frightened at looking unprofessional. By talking about what you need and want, you can help us to be normal, to relax a bit, and to open up.

Next, we're going step back and take a broader look at what's often going on in the lives of those caring for you. Understanding them and their lives should help you appreciate them better. Our first example in sad Lisa, one of the most talented nurses I worked with.

20. Sad Lisa

When I wrote about Pala, so alone and helpless, I mentioned how some head nurses, obsessed as they are with efficiency, make it difficult for staff to be kind. That's why I suggested that you show a little sympathy if your nurse seems emotionally drained. She's helping you, so help her.

But there are also situations where a nurse's sadness has nothing to do with the hospital. The problem may be in her personal life, and a nurse in that situation needs your kindness just as much.

Lisa's Troubles

Petite and pretty, with lovely, long light-brown hair, Lisa was one of my favorite nurses. Were I sick and in a hospital, she'd be one of those I'd most like to have caring for me. And no, she wasn't the sort who'd rush into a room, extruding chattiness like I nurse I once dated, as fun as that can be. She was the quiet, capable type, totally focused on doing her job well. She took her work seriously and thought about everything she did. In *Nights with Leukemia,* she's the one who was prepared to act when a doctor's foolish order to give a cystic fibrosis patient (Kay) vitamin K by IV instead of the girl's usual vitamin pill went bad, triggering a potentially fatal reaction. If you were sick, you'd be very fortunate to have her caring for you.

Lisa was also very much a woman. That was obvious during a visit from a teen-unit nurse who was on maternity leave. The latter had grown so big during her last few weeks on the job, that I joked to myself that she was waiting until eight months, three weeks, six days and some hours into her pregnancy to leave us. A few weeks after the happy event, she dropped by to show off her cute new baby. Lisa was so eager to hold that baby, I could tell she wanted one of her own.

A couple of months later, while Lisa and I were working together, she hinted that she was now pregnant. "She wants a baby," I thought. A few weeks later, wondering why that hint hadn't become a baby announcement, I asked her what had happened. Sadly, she told me that her pregnancy had been "vetoed"—a strange comment and one that made me suspect her husband had forced her to get an abortion.

A few days later, she had more bad news. She'd left her husband, she said, because he was a "little boy," who refused "to grow up" and didn't want a baby because it would take money away from "his toys." This guy, I thought, is a fool for letting someone as wonderful as her get away.

That sad news came near the end of my time at the hospital. I only saw her once after I left. I lived near the hospital and was out walking when she drove past headed for work. She waved, trying to smile, but I could tell she was unhappy. Knowing her well, I knew that, as sad as she was, she was swallowing her pain to give her teen patients the best possible care. She was that kind of nurse.

I brought up Lisa to make an important point. Never forget that the nurses who care for you aren't robots who get wheeled into a closet and plugged into a charger when they go off-duty. They're people just like you, and they have lives outside the hospital that can be as filled with pain as your own. So don't take it personally if a nurse seems distracted and be careful about complaining to the administration over something petty. Your nurse may be lugging around a big bag of hurt. Instead, be kind and considerate. She'll appreciate that and maybe give you special attention. When you're in the hospital, that's good.

A Hospital in a Storm

Lisa's troubles did not end with her baby and marriage woes. In the months just after I left the hospital, her sufferings grew far beyond her private life. She and the hospital's nurses had to cope with a soul-crushing crisis that I'd sensed coming and later heard about from others. The hospital's chaplain—a likable "Mr. Rogers" sort of guy—told me the details when I ran into him a few months later. He began by telling me that the hospital had lost fully twenty percent of its nurses—about one every single weekday—and was finding it impossible to replace them. The nursing administration and nurses were at war, he said. Mandated overtime to cover the vacancies meant nurses were overworked and tired.

That wasn't good. Caring nurses such as Lisa would be frustrated that their patients were being put at risk by angry, tense, overworked staff. Some would leave. Others would hang in there, depressed and exhausted but doing their best to protect the kids from this bureaucratic madness. Still other nurses, those focused on careers and benefits rather than patients, would be outraged that their nursing contract was being violated by too much overtime. They'd not only be angry, they do their best to feed the anger. I was glad I'd left just in time and had not opted to work weekends.

Will you be able to tell if that's happening at your hospital? Since you don't work there, probably not. I'd been working at mine for over two years, and it still took time for me to understand what was going on.

If the morale at your hospital seems low, something like that could be happening. Some hospitals are badly run and have chronically poor staff morale while others, usually well-run, have short episodes like that I saw. In most cases, you may not be able to tell if the nurses taking care of you are dealing with personal issues (Lisa's baby wish) or whether the unit you're on has morale problems, such as staff clashing with the administration. You'll just notice that they seem stressed out or depressed.

What should you do? Focus on cheering them up with smiles and praise. Remember, they need you almost as much as you need them. The better you make them feel, the better your care.

Finally, I hope you never find yourself in a hospital that's going through that much trouble, but if you do, take hope. Everything I suggested when I wrote about Binky still applies. If you're liked by staff, they'll help you negotiate a storm that you, as a patient, have little chance of understanding. They'll look out for you in the storm.

21. SHY ELSIE

A good nickname for this particular nurse might be Miss Matchmaker. She was the daughter of a physician and one of the teen unit's best nurses. One afternoon in late summer, perhaps a month or so after the last Post-Op Girl had left, I began to suspect that she was playing matchmaker between me and the lovely Elsie, a medical technician who visited us several times a day.

Medical technicians were the hospital's unsung heroes. They came, had the grim duty of doing a blood draw no patient enjoyed, and then hurried on. They were almost invisible and never a topic of conversation, which is why I wondered if Miss Matchmaker, in her eagerness to chat with me about Elsie, was trying to get the two of us together.

I also wondered if Elsie might be encouraging her. Perhaps she'd been asking Miss Matchmaker about me. At least twice that summer I'd turned around to find that Elsie had quietly slipped into the room. Both times, I could not shake the feeling that she'd been looking at me just a moment before. "No, that can't be," I told myself. "There's no way I could be that fortunate."

Hospital Gowns and Other Embarrassments

Elsie was easily one of the prettiest girls in a hospital with an abundance of such girls. She was a petite and athletic, with light brown hair, marvelously lovely eyes and a meltingly beautiful smile. Far more important to me, her way with patients told me that she was gentle and kind. There was also something about her that made me believe she was both smart and serious about life—things I like. Knowing her would never grow dull.

First Date Phobia

Alas, all that caught me in the most terrible and dreadful of binds. Call it First Date Phobia. I had it bad. It was narrow in scope but utterly paralyzing. I was absolutely terrified of asking girls I hardly knew out on a first date. Friends I dated all the time. Nurses at the hospital who took the initiative to start a relationship gave me no problem, although I never got serious. I wasn't afraid of girls, I was just absolutely terrified of initiating a first date with a girl I hardly knew. There was a reason why. It was the worst trauma of my entire life, bar none.

It happened shortly before I began work at the hospital. I asked out a girl from church that I hardly knew for no more reason than that she had lovely green eyes. At the time, she seemed to be one of the most have-my-life-together girls I'd ever known. We went to a movie and afterward to her apartment for tea.

There she said that what she was telling me—a guy she'd talked with for maybe a half-hour in total before that evening—was something she was not telling any of her family or friends. In her late twenties, she was in the mother of all "I'll never marry" panics. She was angry at God, angry at men, angry at life, and intent on doing whatever it took to wreck her life completely and utterly. I was even afraid, in the midst of all that mad fury, she'd kill herself.

If she'd been an old friend, I'd have already liked her, and that would have given me the motivation to help. I'd have also had confidence that she'd listen to my advice. Neither was true. I hardly knew her. What I wanted more than anything else was to run away just as fast and far as I could. I hated feeling responsible for her life. Worst of all, I was afraid that, despite my best efforts, she might do something terrible to herself.

I've been through a lot in my life, including almost getting crushed by a tumbling boulder the size of a small car while mountain climbing and having a deranged alcoholic threaten me with a razor-sharp case cutter in Alaska when I worked at a homeless shelter. None created the slightest ripple in my psyche. My mind had calmly decided, "Well, you didn't die, so why fret about it." But this girl's plight affected me far differently. A short story may help you understand.

Imagine yourself crossing a tall bridge on a foggy night. Suddenly, looming out of the darkness in front of you is a young woman who has climbed over the railing and is about to plunge into the cold water far below. Just as she releases her grip on the railing, she sees you and reaches out. You grab her hand and find yourself being pulled over the railing after her. You're terrified that, if you don't let go, you'll be dragged to your death. But you also know that, if you let her go, she'll die.

That was the situation I was in and it lasted for six long weeks. True, I wasn't in any literal danger of dying. I'm not the suicidal type. But in a terrible process psychologists call "transference," all her fears, angers and frustrations had been transferred to me, and they were ripping me apart. Having bound myself that closely to her, I felt utterly trapped. That was terrifying, and it went on and on and on.

The good news is that, with a some fumbling but well-meant help from me, she recovered, later meeting and marrying a wonderful guy, and thus ending her lonely spinster fears. But that experience became my one-and-only PTSD (Post Traumatic Stress Disorder), flashbacks and all.

That, in turn, led to First Date Phobia. If someone as seemingly together as she was could prove such an emotional basket case, I felt, no girl was safe. And yes, I know, that was stupid. What had happened was one in ten thousand. It almost certainly wouldn't happen again. But that did me no good. I had this fear, and I had it bad. The only good news is that my mind had done a good job of walling off the problem to situations that were almost identical to hers—a first date with a seemingly together girl whose situation in life I didn't know.

Putting Life On Hold

In any other set of circumstances, I'd have gotten over those fears quickly. But not long after that I starting working on Hem-Onc. Every night, when I went to work, I had to face situations not that different from that terrifying relationship—situations fraught with the possibility that one blunder on my part might mean someone's death. Every few months, one of the children I liked would die.

To make matters still worse, three months after I began work on Hem-Onc, every one of its experienced night nurses left to be replaced by nurses just out of school who were soon floundering badly. As with that girl who'd decided to trust me on our first date, everyone—nurses on other shifts and parents—turned to me to keep things from falling apart. Again, I was being trusted with what seemed to be an almost impossible task. I had to not only do my job, I had to keep my nurse from botching up hers.

Yes, I coped with that well, but at a serious cost. I focused my attention completely on those kids and didn't take on any issues in my personal life, particularly that dread First Date Phobia. Outside work, I became a bore, living without adventure or change—other than a move to live closer to the hospital. Some day when my life was less stressful, I told myself, I would get rid of that crazy fear, but not now. For now, those kids need me.

Alas, with Elsie that time was now. The more I found out about her, the more I liked her. In my two years at the hospital, I met dozens of single women. She was the only one who stirred my interest. When Miss Matchmaker mentioned that Elsie had been chosen as an amateur model for a major recreational clothing retailer—did I say she was both pretty and athletic—I got their catalog.

The next time Elsie came by the teen unit I mentioned, ever so clumsily, having seen her in the catalog. She turned pink with embarrassment. I was amazed. I didn't know girls could still blush. It took me a few seconds to understand why. One of the pictures showed her and several other girls posing in sport bras. A sport bra is, of course, more like a modest swimsuit top than underclothing. Now I was most charmed. Surrounded by nurses who were so blasé about undressed teen girls, I was delighted to find someone shy and modest.

Our Last Meeting

Alas, despite my rapidly growing interest in her, I was still trapped in that dread First Date Phobia. Then late one summer afternoon Elsie entered the room where I was working and came up to me. Medical technicians were expected to stay on the move, not dallying anywhere. And yet there she was, risking censure and apparently on the unit just to talk with me. Talking fast and almost exploding with interest, she asked me a series of personal questions, including whether I was married or had ever been married.

To this day, I don't know how I seemed to her. Sometimes, in really upsetting situations, I look exactly the opposite of how I feel. Perhaps in my panic and confusion, I looked calm and collected. In reality, I was torn apart. I liked her and she seemed to like me. I wanted to ask her out but couldn't.

I felt like screaming. No other phobia had ever controlled me this way and none probably ever will. I'm afraid of heights, but that didn't keep me from climbing where one slip meant a deadly fall. In those situations I stayed calmed and collected, even when I looked down. Why couldn't I overcome this simple hang up? If chopping off a hand would have cured it, I'd have done that eagerly. But there I stood, frozen and unable to act.

All it would have taken was for one of us to blurt out a suggestion that we have lunch together and things would have also certainly clicked. That first date passed and her lack of a major life crisis assured, I could behave normally. And yet nothing happened. She was shy. I was afraid. After she left, I told myself that, at whatever cost, I needed to act. But could I? I didn't know.

There would be no next time. A few days later Miss Matchmaker gave me the bad news. Elsie was every bit as smart as I'd suspected. She had moved back east to start medical school. Our hurried conversation had been her last, desperate bid to get my attention. She had my attention in spades, but it was too late for both of us.

I hope both Lisa's sorrows about her lost baby and my sadly missed romance with the wonderful Elsie help you to understand something important. When you're in a hospital, don't forget that those who are caring for you may have troubles of their own. They may even be sacrificing something in their personal lives to keep their attention sharply focused on you. So be sure you like them, appreciate what they do for you, and be kind to them.

Now we'll turn our attention back to you and explain some practical steps you can take to prepare for your hospital visit.

22. Preparing Ahead

As we've seen, Heidi and the Twins were pros. They knew how to handle their care and get what they wanted. But as I saw all too often working with teens, when patients first set foot in a hospital, many aren't assertive enough, especially if their illness is a serious one. Only over time do they learn that their visits can be more enjoyable if they take charge of what matters to them. But you don't have to visit

Hospital Gowns and Other Embarrassments

a hospital over and over to learn that skill. Even on your first visit, you can benefit from preparing ahead. A day or two of planning can make a big difference.

1. Have a Go-to Person

First and most important, have a go-to person (or persons) ready. If you can deal with a problem yourself, that's usually better. But remember, if you are unwell enough to be in a hospital, you're likely to be either yucky sick or woozily recovering from some gosh-awful treatment. Getting help under those conditions isn't a sign of weakness. It's being smart.

Going home only a few hours after my hernia operation meant I didn't have to deal with hospital care, but if I had, I'd have been in poor shape to look out for myself. The painkiller I was prescribed gave me the attention span of gnat. I hated not being able to think straight and quickly abandoned it, figuring the pain was better. The four days of constipation that followed the surgery left me feeling so rotten, I didn't want to eat and had trouble sleeping.

Being at home, I didn't need to deal with hospital care. But if I had, I'm not sure how I'd have handled the hassles. Since I'm not the type to yell, I would have probably just gritted my teeth and endured any troubles that came up. I don't want that for you, so have that go-to person lined up before you go, someone to handle situations you're not up to dealing with yourself.

Who you choose depends on the situation. Your mom or dad might be a great choice, particularly since they have legal rights the hospital will recognize. So would a relative or family friend who has a medical or nursing background. If there's an issue in your care, they'll know how to talk with staff.

You might also want to draw in a school-aged friend, a brother, or a sister. Some people have a knack for making things happen, and some don't. If you're in the latter category, but know someone in the former, they can be a big plus. For the little, niggling things, a girl friend might be your best choice. If you're stuck with an obnoxious roommate, for instance, she can visit, see your problem firsthand, and talk to your nurse about it. That'll let you play good cop (patiently suffering) to her bad cop (complaining on your behalf). Patients aren't usually moved, but you might be an exception.

2. Get a Doctor's Orders

Second, think seriously about sharing any concerns you have in advance with the doctor who's handling your care, either the primary physician who refers you to the hospital or the attending physician who takes care of you while there. He or she can write up orders that become part of your treatment—instructions that will be read and followed by your doctors and nurses. Frightened, sensitive little Min is an excellent example of someone who'd have benefited from a firm medical order to not to do anything that might embarrass her. If you have serious concerns that could be covered by such an order, talk with your doctor in advance.

For instance, if you're like the young nurse I mentioned earlier—the one who at the age of twelve spent several days in a hospital having larger and larger sizes of tubing inserted into her urethra—you probably don't want every Tom, Dick and Harry coming by and giving you an under-the-sheets inspection, so a "Females Only" order makes perfect sense. If the hospital or your doctor have never issued orders like that before, then good for them. You'll make the first time. First times are good for hospitals—especially when the issue is embarrassment.

3. Set Conditions in Advance

Third, you may want to anticipate problems by setting conditions on your care, either before you're admitted or on admission. If you'll be at a teaching hospital, the broad exclusions you might adopt include "No Students" and "No Residents." Check with the hospital to see if there are others.

The chief problem you're going to face is that hospitals typically accept these restrictions under the assumption that a patient feels that those in training make more mistakes. If your main concern is with invasions of your privacy, there's not going to be a good match between what you want and what the hospital offers.

"No students" means you won't become an undressed exhibit for prowling bands of knuckle-dragging male medical students—a most worthy goal. If privacy is your primary concern, you might want to opt for that.

But keep in mind that a student, either in nursing or medical school, may be a big plus. Not all are cave men. He or she is likely to give you more time and attention than anyone else. If you value attention, there are benefits to being a nursing student's sole patient for an entire day, and the same can be true of medical students. When I had my car accident, I received lots of attention from the emergency room staff until they realized I wasn't going to die, after which they left to find someone more exciting. From that point on, the only person caring for me was a medical student, who patiently stitched up my two cuts and made sure I got the necessary x-rays. Both nursing and medical students can be a plus, giving you more attention than anyone else, so don't reject them without a lot of thought.

"No residents" means that your care won't be handled by young doctors who've finished medical school and are now getting hands-on training in a particular area. They're still learning and their experience can vary from mere days to several years. Again, you may want to think twice about that exclusion, since at many hospitals that means any issues that come up will have to be taken to the attending physician, and that almost always means a delay. Although I can gripe about residents as well as anyone who has worked at a teaching hospital, it's also true that not only do they get it right almost all the time, they're usually following your case more closely and may be better situated to make the right decision than a more experienced attending physician who is less well-informed about you because he has a hundred other responsibilities.

Whether you want to exclude students and residents also depends on why you're in the hospital. If you're getting surgery on your elbow, you could probably care less how many residents come by to inspect it and test your range of motion. You may even enjoy all the extra attention and—who knows—some of them might prove interesting. But if your care is in a more private area, you may prefer not to be the subject of some stranger's fumbling, bumbling learning process. Just keep in mind that you can have students and residents caring for you and still set specific restrictions on what they do. Medical care requires your consent. More on that later.

4. Discuss and Record

Fourth, be ready just in case something awful happens. Write down what's happening in a handwritten diary or on a cell phone. If you are in a multi-bed room, talk with the other girls. Keep your mom informed about what's going on from the start, particularly if it involves a creepy guy and not just green-tinted mystery meat. The earlier she knows, the easier it will be for her to back you up. Parents dislike teen drama. What you don't want to do is call her, crying and upset, after everything has fallen apart. Adults find a crisis easier to handle if they've been involved from start and are part of the decision-making that leads up to it. Doing that isn't being 'a little girl.' It's grown up and mature.

Technology can help. If you can—even if you have to borrow one—have a cell phone beside your bed with a charger (although perhaps not one so nice it gets stolen). Talking about problems may not always be the best approach, since others can overhear. So text your mom when something happens, giving details. You'll not only be keeping her informed, you'll be creating a time-stamped chain of evidence that's likely to become in handy if this degenerates into dreadful 'he said, she said' mess. That's particularly true if lawyers get involved. We'll discuss that in more detail later.

Also, keep in mind that witnesses may become important. If there's a creep on staff who is lingering a bit too long in a room you share with other girls, when he leaves, say something like, "Did you see that? He needed to be here for about two minutes but he stayed, stalling around, for five. And I don't like the way he kept looking around at us." Your roommates may not be as observant as you, but that will fix what happened in their minds. They'll remember it later.

5. Nurses as Friends

Finally, don't fret that your nurses will be irritated by any special conditions you set on your care. Most like having additional details to chat about at report, and many, if they are women, will enjoy being able to do something that the male residents—normally the ones giving them the orders—can't do.

In fact, in some hospitals, one of the main tensions lies between men (as doctors) who give orders and women (as nurses) who are less than impressed with some of those orders. I wasn't immune to that power struggle myself.

Nor should you overly worry about hurting the feelings of staff guys, and I say that as someone who was one. Your comfort—something you have every right to define—should be a part of proper, professional care. The good sort of guys will be glad to do what it takes to make you comfortable. The bad sort are best kept far away. I'll say more about both later.

Next we talk about sensible ways to dress in a hospital, starting with than pesky gown. Think positive. It isn't as bad as it seems. You can learn to manage it with finesse. You may even grow to like it. It does have some advantages.

23. That Gown

I forget precisely the reason, but I must have been teaching a CPR class at the hospital that morning because, instead of being snug in bed by 7:45, several hours later I returned to medical unit where I was still working nights. Seeing me, the head nurse pounced, her fangs exposed and her claws drawn.

Why, she wanted to know, had I left a patient's gown and sheets soiled when I'd left work that morning? Alas, I couldn't say. As usual, I checked on all my Hem-Onc patients at the end of the shift and everyone, including that Daniel, a boy of about eight, was fine. I suspected she gone off half-cocked, launching an attack without investigating. She often did that.

That night, I asked the nurse I'd been working with if she knew what happened. She had a ready explanation. She'd been in the room when I'd passed through and, after I'd left, she'd shifted Daniel over in his bed. The boy had suction tubing drawing fluid out of his stomach. In the process of moving him, some stomach juices had sprayed out a vent in the tubing and onto his gown and bed sheets. I'd seen nothing in my last check of that child because nothing had yet happened.

Of course, if my nurse had told me, I'd have cleaned it up, but I understood her forgetfulness. Two of the day-shift nurses were as ill-tempered as that head nurse. Creeping up on middle age with unhappy lives, at report they often took their anger out on the younger night nurses. I could understand why my nurse was so panicked at the thought of giving report to them, that she forget to tell me about the spill.

Cleanliness and Comfort

Although what I have just described is an example of dreadful hospital administration that I describe in more detail in *Nights with Leukemia*, it's also an illustration of one trait of good hospitals. They're places where patient cleanliness and comfort matter. It's good that, when patients get soiled, they're cleaned up promptly and not left to lie in their filth. That's something you should be thankful for. Not every hospitalized patient is that fortunate.

That, in turn, is something you should keep in mind when certain difficulties come up with you and that guy staffer who's caring for you. Those cleanliness and comfort issues are also precisely the ones that create the potential for embarrassment, things like changing linen or gowns and being prompt with bedpans. Assistants typically get stuck with the messy stuff.

I know. In *Nights with Leukemia* I describe Josh, the little two-year-old boy that one nurse called the 'Wild Man of Borneo." The first time I saw him, he'd pulled off his diaper and was smearing poop on the rails of his crib. Good hospitals know that staff don't like to clean that up, so they put correspondingly high pressures on them to do it quickly. That includes not just bodily waste but vomiting or spitting up, both common for those helpless and lying on their backs.

A Gown Change

Now suppose, for a moment, that you'd been my patient that morning and that stomach contents spillage had been on your gown rather than Daniel's. Imagine that nurse had told me, as she rushed off to report, that you needed your gown changed. Ah, now we have a problem don't we, particularly if you have little or nothing on under that gown? This has a much greater potential for embarrassment than a mere bedpan. Changing that gown could prove most embarrassing.

Now remember what I said about the pressure on staff to take care cleanliness and comfort issues quickly. If I was taking care of you that morning, I could not say: "Tough luck, young lady. I've been here all night. I'm tired. I want to get home and sleep. You'll just have to put up with that stinky, sticky gown until a day nurse comes around in about fifteen or twenty minutes." Not only would I be behaving like a jerk toward you, when that day nurse found what I'd left for her to do, I'd be in big trouble—and this time legitimately so.

What did I do in those cases? First, I was fortunate because the girls I cared for were trusting and cooperative. Not a single one crossed her arms and said, "You're not taking off my gown, you pervert." That would have been a bit unsettling. With the girl willing, I did my best. I made the entire process as quick and smooth as possible. I had the new gown alongside the girl, so there would be no fumbling. Then I looked her in the eyes and used my peripheral vision to slip off the old and slip on the new. Everything but her face was a blur. They seemed happy with that.

A Secret Technique

But what about you? The guy caring for you might not do what I did. He might take longer than you'd like, and he might not always look into your lovely eyes. As with bedpans and linen changes, is there a less embarrassing approach, and one that you can insist that he follow?

I think there is, but first I should warn you. I've not tested what I'll be suggesting here. As usual, my hospital didn't fret about embarrassing gown changes. I could be as intrusive as I wanted as long as the change got done quickly. I came up with 'look into her eyes' when I cared for Christy and—since other girls also seemed happy with that—I didn't feel any need to improve it. With a thousand other things to worry about, good enough was good enough.

But for you that might not be good enough. You may want something that has real rather than virtual modesty. So here's my as-yet-untested suggestion. First, smile as sweetly as you can. That can work wonders. Then tell this guy you have a 'secret technique' for gown changes that you'd like him to help you with. Remember what I said about Binky. Charm, smiles, and gentle words get you far in hospital where patients are often silent and glum.

The first issue is likely to be the straps at the back of your gown. If they're fastened, either you or he will have to undo them. That's where you might get ready in advance. If you're stuck in bed, fasten only the strap behind your neck. That'll keep the gown from sliding down if you sit up ("Oops!"). You can probably handle that strap yourself.

Next, gowns tend to ride up, so make sure your old gown reaches down far enough before he slips down the sheet. Then comes the awkward part—slipping your arms out of the old gown while still leaving it in place on top of you. If moving around like that isn't easy, he can help by holding the gown steady.

We've now reached the critical step in your 'secret technique.' Have him spread the new gown over you like a camping tent. Hold it up so the old gown doesn't soil the new. Then, with you gripping the new gown, he can slip down the old. Get your arms into the sleeves of the new gown, and hopefully nothing has happened to make you turn even the slightest pink. Afterward, you can smile sweetly and say, "If you like my secret technique, feel free to use it with other girls."

As a guy, my work was made more complicated by the fact that the *more dependent* a girl was on me for everything, the *less likely* she was to have anything on underneath her gown. It was the usual hospital obsession with efficiency. Her clothing changes required assistance. The less she wore, the less work required to change her each day. Changing a gown plus undies was at least twice the work of just changing a gown. As a result, female nurses and assistants dressed those girls in as little as possible. That doesn't have to be. If you'd rather have more on, simply insist on it. They won't mind, and it'll only take a few seconds.

Finally, you're not limited to what I suggest. Come up with your own techniques. If you can handle the gown yourself, say: "Oh, you must be busy. Just bring me a new gown and a wash towel, and I'll change myself." Since you're saving them time, they won't mind at all. Remember, they can't ask you to do that, since that would be shirking work. But if you offer to do it yourself, that's fine.

Getting About

Hopefully, you won't be stuck flat on your back and helpless during your entire hospital stay, so I should say something about what you should do with that gown once you can get up and leave your room, either for a medical procedure or just a change of scenery.

Your biggest problem with that gown usually lies in the back—that revealing slit which opens widely with each step you take. For all the casualness my nurses had about undress in the girls room, they were strictly against girls walking about the halls with the back of their gowns flopping open, entertaining our teen boys. One nurse called that "inappropriate." She would chase the girl down and pin that offending gown up. Like I said, at least we protected our girls from the eyes of boys.

As a good assistant, I did the same, even keeping safety pins in my tunic pocket for just that purpose. But if you'd rather not have a staff guy doing the pinning, do it yourself or get another girl to help. Use two safety pins, one about waist high and the other some six inches below that. Even more important, overlap the two sides of the gown about four inches or more before you pin them together. Given how awful the gown looks, I can't promise that you'll look like an elegant fashion model, but tightening it around the waist will make you look a little less like a giant cotton bag with feet.

On more thing. While I've been critical of how embarrassing a gown with a slit can be, it's also true that almost any other way of dressing patients would be worse. Without that slit, checking a surgery site on your tummy would mean exposing everything from your toes to well above your belly button. And think about it for a moment—without that slit, bedpans would terribly awkward. Used right, a gown with a slit allows staff to do what they must with the least exposure. You just need to make sure that gown is used properly and take care with what you wear underneath. What's beneath that gown is our next topic.

24. Beneath that Gown

As a hospital employee, I could attend medical conferences held at the hospital for free. So when one being held on a Saturday morning for doctors who treated children with major disabilities I went. Quite a few of the kids I cared for had disabilities, so I might learn something useful.

These mostly middle-aged men certainly weren't making much money. The kids they cared for needed lots of attention and their parents were rarely rich. I could see that in the suits they wore. At most medical conferences, the doctors wear expensively tailored suits that say, "I'm a success in my speciality. You should refer patients to me." These child disability specialists were wearing suits that might have come from the bargain rack at J. C. Penneys. They were dedicated to their kids and not in it for the money. I was impressed.

Differing Twins

Something happened that day, however, that you might want to think about. One doctor took the stage to describe two patients of his who were twins and yet had very different medical conditions. One was quite normal, and indeed she was a pretty sixteen-year-old girl. The other was so severely disabled, she could barely stand and then only hunched over. The difference, he said, existed from before they were born, but wasn't genetic. In the womb, the placenta of the healthy girl had implanted itself normally, while that of the other girl had placed itself on top of her sister's, resulting in much less nutrition. To show the difference between the two, he displayed a picture of the two girls, with the healthy teen doing her best to hold up her much smaller sister. Two things struck me as I looked at the picture.

The first was sadness. I wondered how that healthy twin must have felt seeing her sister every day and knowing that her own good health had been bought at the expense of her sister's crippling disabilities. Did she feel guilty, or did she focus on doing all she could for that sister. The doctor didn't say.

The other thing that struck me was her willingness to be photographed alongside her sister clad only in underwear. Did she know when she posed for that picture that she was agreeing to have it shown to the hundred or more doctors who were there that day and perhaps published in a medical journal or textbook read by thousands? I'm not sure she did.

She probably thought it would just go into her sister's medical file and agree to help a sister she loved.

Passive Modesty

Her story illustrates something I wondered about as I cared for these adorable teen girls. What most practiced was passive modesty. They adjusted how they dressed as little as possible for hospital life. That healthy sixteen-year-old twin is a good example. Probably every year since she was a small child, her picture had been taken alongside her sister to create a medical record. A two-piece swimsuit would have documented the changes just as well, and yet she still showed up with undies on. That's passive modesty. It does as little as possible, not thinking ahead or looking for an alternative. Perhaps she didn't care. But most of the girls certainly seemed to care about that, and yet most still took little concrete action to prevent it. Look at how they dressed.

First, they almost never worn bras. No, I didn't peek. That was easy enough to see, given the open slit in the back of their gowns. Most of the time that was sensible. In those shapeless gown, all these girls had the figure of cotton blobs. Going braless didn't lead to embarrassment either, since that's one area the gown covers well.

But most cases aren't every case. Remember Ginny and her regular central line care? Her embarrassment came because it only took a few seconds for that nurse to loosen her gown's top string and leave her bare to the waist. "Eek!," she must have thought. At that moment, I imagine she wished she had a bit more on, particularly with me busily working across the room. But notice that she wasn't asserting her right to avoid being embarrassed, either by what she wore under that gown or what she expected of her nurse. Her modesty was certainly real and intensely emotional. I could see that in her eyes when I turned around. But it was also passive. That's the problem in a nutshell, and that's where you may want to be more assertive.

Second, with their underpants the girls showed a similar passive modesty. Most did wear panties, and earlier I did my best to convince you to do likewise. But more than that is needed. If you're going to move about the halls, rest assured, given the looseness of that gown, those undies will show. Bed linen changes mean flashing them yet again, and that's also true if you hop from your bed to a gurney to be taken down hallways filled with gawking strangers who may also get a peek if you're not careful—and it's hard to be careful when you are sick or fretting about an upcoming medical exam.

Yes, that gown certainly makes those exams easy, but it also does a poor job of covering you. Unfortunately, you will have to live with it. Hospitals aren't going to adopt six layers of neck-to-ankle coveralls with locked zippers as their preferred attire. Nor would they be happy if you showed up dressed that way. But, as we will see, there are things you can do that won't upset staff.

After Your Surgery

We'll start with a situation that may fit you. Moving about in bed or inside the hospital means some exposure, but the situations that lead to the most embarrassments usually come after an operation. Quite a few surgeries mean sutures on your tummy because there's a lot in there to fix. To check those sutures, an assortment of people, some total strangers, will suddenly appear and yank your gown aside.

I confess. I was one of those dastardly gown yankers. If you'd been a patient of mine, for a couple of days after your surgery, the first time I came around in the morning I'd check that place on your tummy (or wherever) for either evidence of bleeding or a redness that might mean infection. That's not something I could skip.

Yes, I was a well-behaved boy, taking care to show as little as possible. But there was nothing to make me behave that way, certainly no hospital policy. If a guy came up to your bed and flipped your gown halfway to your face, showing—for all the world to see—those embarrassingly tiny bikini panties with the dancing bunnies, any complaint you might make would get you nowhere. He was 'just doing his job,' the hospital would say. No, I don't believe he was either. Nor do I think he just wanted a peek at the cute bunnies.

The problem doesn't end there. Post-surgery inspections aren't just visual. There'll be a lot of touching too. After your surgery, hospitals are likely to thump, listen or poke your chest and tummy. Mysterious as that may seem, it really is necessary.

- Thumping your chest and back makes sure your lungs aren't filling up with fluid, which would be very bad. What they are doing is a bit like thumping a watermelon, where a hollow sound means ripeness. You want your lungs ripe and full of air.

- Listening to your tummy ensures that you have normal bowel sounds, meaning pops and gurgles. When I had my hernia surgery, my bowels rebelled and shut down for several days. They needed time to recover. The same could happen to you. Surgeons need to know what your bowels are doing.

- Poking on your tummy and asking how that feels can tell a doctor much about what's going on inside you. Grin and bear it.

Preparing for Inspections

The downside of all that thumping, listening and poking is that your gown gets moved this way and that, leaving you woefully dependent on what you are wearing underneath. Remember Ginny. If she had been wearing something on top, she wouldn't have been embarrassed when I turned around. She could have smiled. You want to be able to smile too.

What can you do? Wearing a bra all the time would be uncomfortable, especially when you're sick. But there's no reason why you can't have an easy-to-slip-on bra, a sports bra, or even swimsuit top by your bed to put on should the need arises. There are even paper bras you can order online. Since you're young, almost every time someone has a legitimate medical reason for dropping down your gown, they're not checking your breasts. Cover up and you can smile as that slightly creepy resident thumps and listens for way too long to your chest or tummy with his icy stethoscope and cold hands.

It's also good to decide in advance what underpants you'll wear. Your own feelings should be your guide. Ask yourself if it would bother you if a half-dozen interns, residents, or a staff guy see what you're wearing. If the answer is yes, then change what you wear. It's that simple. Within the limits of the hospital's rules, take charge of your under-thingies.

If the thought of being seen in those tiny dancing-bunny panties doesn't bother you any more than being seen in a swimsuit bikini, then that's fine. But if it does, wear something that covers a bit better. If being seen in the baggy, unsexy, 'granny' underpants that the hospital provides is all right, then wear those. You'll save yourself the hassle losing your clothes in the hospital wash and, by being bland, you'll attract less attention from the wrong guys. As always, find your own balance between convenience and modesty.

Most important of all, if being seen in any sort of underwear is more than you'd like, substitute outerwear such as swim tops and gym shorts. No, the staff isn't going to get upset over that. Swim tops won't interfere with what they need to do, and gym shorts are as easy to slip down for bedpans as undies, which is all that matters. In fact, with a swimsuit top and gym shorts on, you can relax and do cartwheels or twirl down the hall like a Russian ballerina—assuming you feel up to that. Gym shorts have another plus. Your favorite panties may end up lost forever in the hospital wash, but staff won't make that mistake with gym shorts.

No, the staff isn't going to laugh if you dress like a gym class. True, during my ten months of caring for teen girls, I never saw one in gym clothes. It was either underclothes or nothing. But if one had dressed that way, I'd have thought, "That's smart. More girls should do that. It'll make them more comfortable and my work less complicated."

More Suggestions

Wearing swimsuit tops and gym shorts also has another plus. It signals to nurses that you're not 'into' being exposed to every passing staff guy. That's a lesson some need to learn. Remember, these nurses aren't being intentionally cruel. They just see a lot of nudity and, thanks to their training, believe it's no big deal, especially the guy-see-girl sort. Make clear you're an exception, and most will treat you differently. You won't even have to say anything.

If the hospital allows it, bring your own pajamas and a bathrobe, wearing them at night as soon as your nurse says that's OK. Wearing pajamas will encourage you to change to street clothes in the morning. That's good because, the more you dress like home, the better you'll feel.

Doctors often don't let you know when they'll drop by. If you aren't properly dressed, top and bottom, when they arrive, ask them to step outside the curtain while you change. (If they have male medical students in tow, be extra firm.) That'll teach them patience, which is good for their doctorly souls. No one needs to learn patience more than they.

If a situation arises when you fear that your gown will be flipped much too high, perhaps in front of a half-dozen medical students, set firm limits. Position an arm so the gown can only be pealed from one side or move aside the gown yourself just enough to show what needs to be seen. Use body language to say, "this far and no further."

In short, display an active rather than a passive modesty. If you want something, make it happen. That gown offers little protection, so wear something underneath that you don't mind showing. I promise you, hospitals don't consider that a crime. You won't have to appear before the dread Board of Mandated Patient Indecency. There is no such board.

I've already talked about nurses, assistants, and other staff you're likely to encounter in a hospital. Now I'll explain doctors from the most senior specialists to the newest residents in training.

25. Understanding Doctors

S ometimes, an expert in an area would be scheduled to talk in one of the small conference rooms near the cafeteria. Staff like me—I still working nights—could grab a breakfast tray and join. This particular morning, an infectious disease expert was to speak, so I decided to delay my bedtime, figuring I could set my alarm for a bit later in the afternoon.

Senior Specialists

I was glad I did. Two of the nation's top Hem-Onc specialists sat down next to me, men so high above me in the hospital's pecking order, I'd never met them personally. They and I were there for precisely the same reason. Chemotherapy blew away the immune system of our children, leaving them open to lethal infections. That created a problem: "When all I know is that a child is running a fever," one of them asked, "how can I know which antibiotics to prescribe?"

That was a good question, and one for which the infectious disease expert had no easy answer. I left appreciating just how difficult it was for our Hem-Onc specialists to make life-or-death decisions. All these two men could do was make an educated guess and hope that one of the antibiotics they chose was the right one. It was like making a shot in the dark except that, if he missed, a child might die.

Remember that, especially if you're sick with some terrible disease and have highly trained specialists caring for you. You'll probably find that they're skilled at treating your disease and at formally interacting with you as a patient. Any question you ask, they'll have a ready answer. If they weren't good, they wouldn't have risen to the top. But the flip side is that they've invested many years of their lives in becoming good in one narrow speciality, one that often means life-or-death for their patients. That means something you should not forget.

That narrowness spells danger for a specialist. Compared to them, I was safe. I could like those delightful Hem-Onc kids, knowing that, if I burned out over a child's death, I could do something else with my life. These specialists don't have that freedom. Year after year, they must continue to treat their patients, knowing some will die. At the time I worked on Hem-Onc, almost one third of our children died. Today the numbers are better, but it's still about one in five.

Ask yourself how would you feel if, each year, one in five of your friends died. Before long, you might find it painful to make new friends. Rather than suffer that hurt, you'd withdraw, having few or no friends. That's the problem these specialists face with their patients.

That's why you're likely find that, although they can be reassuring and will give you top-notch care, they often show professional detachment. They won't really get close to you. Don't let that bother you. It's not because they don't care. It's because they must guard themselves from getting too personally involved. Even the nurses I worked with on Hem-Onc talked about that problem, and it's far easier for a nurse to move on than a pediatric cancer specialist.

That said, in addition to their great skill, there's one advantage to having them care for you. If you need something special or out-of-the-ordinary done, perhaps something involving embarrassment, they're often the best person to ask. Major hospitals exist because of them. Without them, patients would go elsewhere, so there's no one over them to say, "No, you can't order that." In a hospital, their word is law. Get them on your side, and you'll get what you want.

Physicians in General

How about most other physicians, those who—while they may have a formal speciality (such as pediatrics)—aren't so highly specialized? If your illness is less serious, they're the ones who'll care for you. There, the issues are different.

Kayla illustrates their world. She was a quiet, dark-haired nine-year-old girl whose family physician initially diagnosed her joint pain as juvenile arthritis. After his efforts to treat that failed, he sent her to the arthritis clinic at my hospital, where in a matter of minutes she was transferred to Hem-Onc. Joint pain is one of the symptoms of leukemia, and that's what she actually had.

Was that family doctor incompetent? Probably not. Of all the children he sees, only one in thousands will have leukemia and even fewer will have joint pain as their first symptom. He simply had such an abundance of possibilities, choosing the correct one wasn't easy. He wasn't an expert in either juvenile arthritis or leukemia. What he knew well were the usual childhood illnesses. That's the key difference between these two doctors. One knows a lot about a little. The other knows a little about a lot.

In a much more modest way, I experienced that same difference when I moved from Hem-Onc to the teen unit. On Hem-Onc, I'd become a specialist of sorts. I knew children with leukemia very well. By the time I left, I not only had more experience with those children than any of the night nurses, I had more experience than all three combined. I'd seen almost anything that could happen.

That's because there's an odd sort of simplicity that comes with extreme specialization. A few years ago, some cancer experts hired an expert to study their decision-making process. After following them around for a few weeks, he came to them with his answer. Everything they did, he told them, depended on the answer to some combination of about 120 questions. They were dumbfound. "It can't be that simple," they said, "we have spent years learning to do what we do."

It was and it wasn't. Quite frankly, I'd never want to be treated by a non-specialist simply going by those 120 questions and answers. There's still room for judgment, as well as knowing, based on new research, when one of those 120 Q&As need changing. When I worked on Hem-Onc, its doctors were continually refining had they did. Going with last year's or even last month's answers might mean death for some child.

That said, there's much in medicine that even someone as little-trained as I could grasp. On Hem-Onc, the routine decisions were so predictable, I could have written the medical orders myself. For instance, when an immunosuppressed child spiked a temperature, we'd do a blood draw to find out what his infection was and then give Tylenol to lower his temperature. There were occasions in the middle of the night when my nurse or I told a new resident what to do.

When I moved to the teen unit, I experienced cultural shock. Before, I'd had nothing to do with surgical patients. Now I not only had surgical patients, I had serious ones, along with patients with mental issues such as anorexia. In fact, I had patients with every imaginable disease a teen could have. For our specialists, that wasn't hard. They came, saw their particular patients, and left. For nursing staff like me, it was confusing. I'd left a unit where I felt on top of my job. I'd come to one where many my patients had something new to me.

That's the problem that generalists face. When you go to them with some vague complaint, there might be dozens of diseases that could be responsible, some of them ones they've never seen. They also may not have every fact on the tip of their tongue. As a result, they may stumble around, running one test and then another before they get it right—or at least send you to a specialist who does get it right.

That's why you should cut these generalists a bit of slack. Modern medicine is too much for anyone to know, particularly busy doctors. I've already explained why the nurses who care for you are human. Now I'm saying the same about doctors.

Emotionally, this bewildering array of patients and diseases may make your generalist seem distracted. Since I'm not a doctor, I'll offer an illustration from what I did. Suppose you're one of my patients and new to the hospital. You've decided you want my attention or sympathy. Perhaps it's one of the embarrassment issues we've been discussing. Perhaps it's something else.

Now look at what I am thinking. My nurse that day is ticked off for reasons I can't understand. She and I have already clashed twice. There's a little ten-year-old girl in the next room who's dying of an inoperable brain tumor (a true event). No one in her family ever comes to visit. In my spare moments, I'm wrestling with what we can do for her. To make matters still worse, a spoiled eleven-year-old boy has been loudly complaining that the wiener in his hot dog is green. He's hungry and yelling that he wants meat that doesn't come from a 'mutant animal.'

That's when you approach me with a request that requires some emotional sensitivity on my part. Can I shove all that aside and focus exclusively on you? Maybe, but it won't be easy. It takes time and experience to develop the skill to juggle many things. For that, I need to be able to do some things so well, they become almost automatic. That frees me to focus on other things, including your feelings. If I've dealt with green wieners before, that's one less thing preying on my mind. If I haven't, then that boy leaves me stewing and wanting to tell him to just quit whining and eat the blasted thing.

Emotional issues are especially difficult to juggle. On the medical unit, for instance, our young kids were often frightened to be sick and far from home. Over time, reassuring them and building their trust in me became second nature. I didn't have to think about it. I just did it. On the teen unit, I faced a similar issue winning the trust of teen girls like you, particularly over these embarrassing things. I never got as good as I wanted, but I was getting better, as I'll mention in my last chapter.

The same juggling difficulty affects physicians. In fact, the issues they're wrestling with were far more important than mine. The most serious medical issue I might face was fluid balance—meaning whether a boy was peeing out about the same amount as the fluids he was taking in. You don't have to be a rocket scientist to add up two sets of numbers and compare them. You do have to be very sharp and focused to cope with the complex issues that trouble doctors.

That's why it's good not to expect too much from your doctors. If they get the medicine right and don't treat you badly, that should be enough. Don't expect them to be superhuman, able to read your mind and meet your every need.

Patients as Special

There's something else about doctors that matters—their limited perspective. My nurse and I spend more time with patients like you than doctors, who must juggle dozens of them. As my patient, you'd have been one of maybe ten teenagers over several eight-hour days. For me, you're the cute girl in Bed 3 who always gives me a mischievous smile when I come into your room. You the one who's always reading, always listening to music, or always eager to talk. That makes you special.

On the other hand, a hospital physician, either a specialist or generalist, may only see you for a few minutes every few days. His notes about you are likely to be more real to him than you are. Focused on treating your disease, you're likely to become the X disease in Room Y getting Z treatment. That's not good or bad. That's just reality. Would you rather he remember that you collect butterflies but forget why you're in the hospital? Probably not. You might end up a dead collector of butterflies.

That's why your nurse and I see you differently. It's also why, for the emotional side of your care, it is better to depend on us rather than specialists who are making life-and-death decisions or generalists juggling more details about medicine than their brains were meant to handle. Just be happy that those doctors are giving you good medical care.

Do you get what I'm saying? It isn't easy being a physician. A doctor often makes decisions that can result in life or death for patients. A doctor juggles dozens of medical issues for many dozens of patients. That does not leave much energy for the little things that affect you emotionally—including embarrassment issues. That's unfortunate but true.

That's why, although I hope you have an amiable relationship with your doctors, I suspect you're going to be disappointed if you want more. Be happy for good medical care and look to nursing staff—along with your family and friends—for warmth and emotional support. That's where you'll find friendship.

26. UNDERSTANDING RESIDENTS

There's one final group of physicians that I should introduce to you, because they'll be appearing, with all their potential for perversity, in the next chapter. Keep in mind that they're only likely to be part of your care if you're at what's called a teaching hospital. In general, that means hospitals located in a large city with close ties to medical and nursing schools. If you're seriously sick, they're usually the best places to be. The fact that residents are often working long hours for a pittance, also means that those hospitals can offer more charitable care.

A Learner's Permit

Because residents are usually recent medical school graduates who're learning hands-on medicine, there's a wide range of abilities among them. Someone who's just out of medical school and rotating through a treatment area for a few weeks to get a little exposure will know far less than someone who's spent several years specializing in that sort of care. You can think of the first as someone who has a learner's permit to drive a car. It's perfectly OK to be a bit nervous if you're in the seat beside them.

How can you tell which is which? Hospitals don't want patients to know that. They'd rather you not realize that some of those caring for you are capable of making real doozies of mistakes. From what I have seen, medication dosage errors are particularly likely to come from less experienced residents. They get numbers from a book or screen and, when they misread or miscalculate, there's nothing in their experience to tell them "that's too much."

It's also true that hospitals may have subtle differences in badging or dress, so the staff can tell who's a first year resident (often called an intern), and who is three years into some speciality. The first needs to be watched like a hawk, lest he make a serious mistake, while the second can usually be trusted.

You won't know those differences and will need to look for different clues. Generally, someone who seems confident and knows what they're doing is more experienced, but that's not always true. Some will bluff about things they don't know, particularly if no other medical staff are around to correct them. If they're in a group—residents sometimes travel in packs—it's usually easy to spot who's in charge. Finally, as in any organization, the new residents often get the rotten assignments, including long hours and night shifts.

Male Residents

Elsewhere I explained why you should not expect women, either doctors or nurses, to automatically protect you from being embarrassed. As I pointed out, they're not being mean. It's just that, after the desensitization that's a part of their training, they regard an undressed you as no big deal. The answer is to get through to them, in words and other ways, that you don't like that. Remember, they're not being cruel. They're just doing what they regard as professional.

Now I'm going to look at the male equivalent, which is one that can involve conscious and even calculating cruelty. The good news is that, because this guy behavior is conscious, the kinder residents won't do it. They'll treat you in a most gentlemanly fashion.

The bad news is that many residents are, by training and inclination, little influenced by kindness or gentlemanliness. They don't mean well and may use their hospital position as a cover for something devious. Keep in mind that, while what I describe here might be true of any staff male, there are reasons why male residents pose a particular risk to young women in general and girls your age in particular.

That's because residents float around a hospital, not accountable to anyone other than more senior residents, who are often guys with the same mind set as they. Also, as you will discover in the next chapter, the need to 'train' residents can be used to cover a multitude of perversities.

In contrast, nursing staff are on mostly female teams that work closely together. If I were to get out of line with a girl, the nurse I worked with would almost certainly notice and react much more effectively than she did in the next chapter when that wolf pack of lecherous male residents took advantage of a helpless Carina. There, her protests against what they were doing had little effect.

Imagine for a moment, that I decided to pretend that lovely young Carina not only needed a bath, but needed my manly assistance getting into the tub. As you will discover, Carina would not have protested— that was her core problem. But the nurse I was working with would have almost certainly noticed. She knew as well as I did that Carina needed no help. She'd have raised hell with me and gone to the head nurse, who was my boss as well as hers. For the record, the thought of getting Carina into a bath never came to me. As you'll soon discover, the equivalent behavior for male residents did occur to a host of them.

No Heart for Patients

But the real problem with male residents is more than a lack of accountability. It lies in the failure of medical schools to give their students the heart—meaning proper feelings toward their patients—that all physicians need. I do believe most acquire that heart after a few years in practice, thanks to all the time they spend caring for people. But many of the residents I met had not learned that and that was particularly true in how they treated our teen girls. Put bluntly, they saw those often helpless girls as sex objects rather than people.

A seemingly unrelated incident illustrates where I think the problem lies. Just before my first Christmas at the hospital, one of the Hem-Onc nurses invited me to a party at her apartment. About twenty of the hospital's other staff crowded in, and I wondered why so many of the single nurses seemed eager to talk with me. "I'm just an aide," I thought. "Why aren't they talking with these soon-to-be-rich residents?"

Then I glanced around at the single, male residents at the party and realized that none were fit company. All were drunk. I was disgusted. Both they and I were probably there for the same reason—to meet single nurses outside work. Yet they'd rendered themselves incapable of talking with them. Most pitiful.

That illustrates a point that I heard nurses discussing among themselves. Some of the hospital's residents, high IQ products of four years of college and four more of medical school, seemed woefully lacking in people skills. In the technical intricacies of medicine, they might be sharp. That's what medical school had emphasized. But socially, they were often woefully lacking, particularly with the opposite sex.

That's why they preferred being drunk to talking with a bevy of pretty nurses. You saw the same thing when the resident who'd attempted to do a spinal tap on Pala stalked off without a word of apology to her. He simply didn't know how to sympathize—even for a few seconds—and was too frightened about what his supervisor would say for failing the procedure.

The problem, I believe, lies in the stress that medical school places on facts and technique to the exclusion of almost all else. I say that as someone whose introduction to medicine was the exact opposite. The contrast may help you to understand them.

I Develop a Heart

The full story is in *Nights with Leukemia*, but I'll tell part of it here. After I was hired, the hospital gave me one week of classroom training followed by three weeks of working days on the medical unit. Most of what I did there was busy work—changing sheets and taking temperatures. I was soon bored.

In the southwest corner of the unit, however, was a cluster of seven rooms that made up Hem-Onc. If mine fields and machine guns had been placed at the entrance, it would not have seemed more off limits to me. The sight of pale, emaciated children with only wisps of hair terrified me. I thought, "How could anyone work there?"

Finally, the night came when I began night shift. It was then that I discovered I'd been hired specifically to work Hem-Onc. Those sad, pitiful, terrifying children were now my patients.

At that time, I knew virtually nothing about leukemia or how it was treated. All I knew was what I soon discovered—that those kids needed me to get through those long, scary nights. As a result, I quickly acquired the 'heart' that I fault medical school for not providing its graduates. There was nothing abstract about what I was doing. I knew the feelings of my young patients before I learned the facts about their treatment. I saw frightened kids before I understood their frightful disease. I knew the horrors of chemotherapy before I learned why we inflected so much suffering. In short, I had a heart before I had a head.

It'd be wrong to say I liked the work. I hated leukemia with a passion. I hated the miseries we had to place our children through in order to save them. I hated the fear I saw in their eyes and the hurt in the eyes of their parents. Most of all, I hated the dying. What I liked were the children themselves. What I liked was the opportunity to do all I could for them. What I liked was that, most of the time, we gave them back their lives.

There's an old belief that, when we make choices, those choices shape us. The choice I made was that, in everything I did, those children would get first priority. If they hurt, I'd be there doing everything I could to ease their pain. If they were lonely—and the parents of some children couldn't be there overnight—I'd find the time to rock them to sleep. And perhaps most important of all for the story I'm telling here, I had no blind allegiance to the system of which was a part. I also became the enemy of anything the hospital might do that would harm them.

The last is the key to understanding this book. Liking those kids trumped any desire on my part to fit in with the system. If something was cruel, I would try to change it, despite my lowly position. If something was harming one of my patients, I'd try to stop it, even if that meant risking my job. I believed in what we were doing in general, but secretly I was an occasional rebel.

It was into that world that a few teen girls appeared—particularly Maria, Christy and Tina. The liking for my patients that had driven all my care of Hem-Onc children was transferred to them but with a new complication. With small children, embarrassment was never an issue. With these teen girls it was. Maria had wanted her nurse to take care of that bedpan. She got me instead. The dying Christy already had enough to deal with. Having a guy as her caregiver meant complications. And last but not least was young Tina, desperate to do anything to live.

That attitude only intensified when I found myself on the teen unit and increased even more when I realized that, with most guys so morose and withdrawn, most of my good relationships were going to be with those girls. Liking the children on Hem-Onc, meant I hated the pain of chemotherapy. Liking these girls meant I hated that my routine care might embarrass them.

Now take away that heart and that liking and what do you have left? You have medical residents whose prime motivation is impressing their superiors. They're very much a part of the system. In that narrow world, patients become little more than teaching tools. Failing Pala's spinal tap was failing to learn a procedure, risking censure. It wasn't hurting an already terrified young woman. That's why I suggest that many—although certainly not all—of these residents had yet to develop a heart. Also, don't forget that, while my warnings here focus on residents and new doctors, they apply equally well to older doctors with something wrong inside. Age itself doesn't offer protection.

Add to that the fact that many of these residents were single males in their mid-to-late twenties, and you have a recipe for sex-tinged trouble. These guys had spent too long lingering over medical textbook drawings of female anatomy, perhaps along with illustrations on how to do a pelvic exam. Now they would have an opportunity to do just that on an exceptionally pretty girl—the defenseless young Carina. She illustrates, all too well, the danger I'm warning about. Take what I say seriously, but don't obsess over it. It's unlikely to happen to you. Just be ready to act if it does. Later, I'll explain what to do.

27. Defenseless Carina

I'm not sure how the word spread, but from all over the hospital male residents came to 'learn' how to do a pelvic exam on Carina, a heart-stoppingly pretty fifteen-year-old with lovely light-brown hair. Since only one exam was needed for a pelvic inflammatory disease (PID) diagnosis, after no less that eight of those intimate, probing exams, the nurse put her foot down and ran those lecherous doctors-in-training out of the exam room. She was still ticked off when I came back from lunch.

Pelvic Inflammatory Disease

For those who wonder, this is how the Center for Disease Control defines Carina's PID. It's a dastardly, complication-ridden infection that no sane woman or teen girl wants to get.

Pelvic inflammatory disease (PID) refers to infection of the uterus (womb), fallopian tubes (tubes that carry eggs from the ovaries to the uterus) and other reproductive organs that causes symptoms such as lower abdominal pain. It is a serious complication of some sexually transmitted diseases (STDs), especially chlamydia and gonorrhea. PID can damage the fallopian tubes and tissues in and near the uterus and ovaries. PID can lead to serious consequences including infertility, ectopic pregnancy (a pregnancy in the fallopian tube or elsewhere outside of the womb), abscess formation, and chronic pelvic pain.

Take particular note of some of the possible consequences—never being able to have a child, a life-threatening ectopic pregnancy, and a pain in the gut that never goes away. This isn't a case of the sniffles. It's a highly destructive infection that can completely wreck a girl's entire life while she's still a teen.

The Girl Who Couldn't Say No

It was easy to see how Carina had been lured into the behaviors that led to her infection. I cared for her during her entire stay, and I never met anyone else who seemed to have less of a self in the sense of an ability to say "no." She was passive and easy-going, which no doubt added to her attractiveness to men of all sorts, good and evil. But since that was not balanced by any good sense or a strong will, that softness was making her life a living hell.

In medicine there's a term called 'compliance' that refers to following a doctor's orders. Carina's problem was that she was all compliance and no resistance. That's why she'd gotten her PID from a guy or guys unknown. That's also why she let all those eager young male residents examine her without protest. If you've never had to endure a pelvic exam, here's how the National Cancer Institute describes the procedure. It's no fun at all, especially when done by a series of over-eager guys.

A physical examination in which the health care professional will feel for lumps or changes in the shape of the vagina, cervix, uterus, fallopian tubes, ovaries, and rectum. The health care professional will also use a speculum to open the vagina to look at the cervix and take samples for a Pap test.

Keep in mind that with Carina the embarrassment issues were different from those of any other girl I cared for. With her, the issue wasn't what she regarded as embarrassing or wronging her—which seemed to be almost nothing—but how we as hospital staff should treat her based on what was best for her, which obviously included making sure she never got another PID. We needed to help her acquire the will power to say no. At least that's what we should have done. These most-intrusive exams by eight strange guys weren't helping her learn to say no.

For my part, I found myself liking her. The same fragility and vulnerability that attracted sexual predators made me want to protect her. Each morning, before she left her room, I would catch her and pin up the back of her gown. If I hadn't, she'd have wandered around the unit, her bright red panties—definitely not hospital issue—attracting the attention of teen boys who were best kept away. Like I said, she was all compliance and no resistance. She had no self to say, "Do this" or "Don't do that." None at all.

Look back and recall the other girls I've written about. Pala was overwhelmed by events and needed protecting until she could recover and run her own life again. Tina was in far worse shape. Because of us and our procedures, her girlish spirit had been broken. She was behaving in ways that made no sense for a young girl. In contrast, Carina seemed to have no will of her own to be either overwhelmed by circumstances or broken by mistreatment. I never got the impression that she was being swept off her feet by the guys who were wrecking her life. It was just a matter of what they wanted, they got. That inability to say no was what was so sad about Carina. That's not something I want to happen to you, hence this book. At its heart, this book is about saying no and making it stick. That's true outside as well as inside a hospital.

I'd like to say more here about how badly the hospital treated Carina, but that doesn't fit with the theme of this book, which is helping you cope with your own embarrassing situations. If you're interested in what I have to say about her, look for my short book, *Carina, The Girl Who Couldn't Say No*. As a digital ebook, it'll be free, so it's widely read.

Facing the Unpleasant

Instead, I want to use my experience with Carina to bring up a problem that I hope, above all others, you never have to face during your hospital stay. And yes, I know that you may not enjoy reading what I'll say here. I don't blame you. It is upsetting and even scary. Looking, leering, groping and even molestation and sexual assault aren't pleasant topics, particularly when they're done by those in positions of power in a medical context and even under a medical pretext. They're more than a bit terrifying. But such things do happen in hospitals—even in one for children—as Carina's shabby, 'we are just doing this to learn' treatment proves.

Just keep what I say in balance. What I'll be talking about here is unlikely to happen to you. I cared for hundreds of children and teens during my roughly 26 months at that hospital. This was the only such incident I saw, and it was cut short by a watchful nurse. So if you find yourself frightened by what you read here, remind yourself: "This is rare." And while it's good that you read what I'll be saying here, don't let yourself dwell on it unless events make that necessary.

I should mention something else. People who do these vile things are often excellent judges of feminine weakness and naivety. They know how to spot 'safe' victims. So, if you're the type who has trouble saying no, or if you regularly find yourself pushed into situations you don't like but can't resist, pay special attention to what I say here. You could become a target.

On the other hand, if you're the strong sort, like the Nina I discussed earlier (the girl who wouldn't set aside her blanket to be weighed), you might want to watch out for the girls around you. Like that nurse who looked out for Carina, women should protect one another.

Finally, keep in mind that Carina's case was clear-cut. The motives of the male residents were all too obvious, as that nurse's righteous fury shows. The medical benefits to pretty Carina of those extra 'look-see' exams by drooling doctors-in-training were non-existent. They weren't going to turn up anything that wasn't already known. The training value of the exams—which she was under no obligation to provide—were also virtually nil. Pictures in textbooks would have served almost as well.

If those in charge believed that these residents absolutely had to have 'hands on' experience with sexually transmitted diseases, an afternoon spent at a public health clinic that catered to middle-aged prostitutes would have served better than intruding into the private areas of a highly troubled fifteen-year-old girl. What happened to her was inexcusable.

Now we take up how you can become aware when you're in danger.

28. YOUR FEELINGS MATTER

After I'd been working on Hem-Onc for several months, I began to sense something that would trouble me more than anything else during my entire time at the hospital. Medical orders, I realized, could go terribly wrong. In the middle of the night with limited staff and caring for seven children battered by chemotherapy and fighting a fatal illness, a mistake could quickly turn deadly. Since my main job was to watch over these children, sounding the alarm if something went wrong, I might be a child's last and only hope. I had to listen to any feeling or hunch that a child wasn't right, however subtle.

Following Intuitions

To protect these sick children, I had to handle three problems properly. The first was one I could manage myself. Initially, my intuition that a child was in trouble was little more than a gut-level feeling that might flash through my mind in an instant and be gone. "This child isn't acting normal," I would think. Why is that important? Because the mind is a sensitive instrument and little children rarely hide their feelings. They're not good with words, but changes in their personality or behavior mean a lot. Listening to those hunches was something I could do, although it meant constant vigilance. Every fleeting impression had to be examined, no matter how tired and sleepy I felt.

Enlisting Others

Other people were a necessary part of the second problem, making it more complicated. With them, my problem was being believed. At that time, intuitions carried little weight in a medicine that prided itself on doing things by the numbers. I needed medical reasons for getting a child's medical orders changed. That especially mattered on two nights when I felt a Hem-Onc child was in serious trouble.

The first came when I was holding Olivia, a little two-year-old girl with leukemia, so her mother could take a short break. As soon as the troubling thoughts came, I tripped the call light to bring my nurse. Then I sat down to come up with a medical reason for stopping the chemotherapy, which had already run past its allotted 24 hours. Yes, I should have found a reason before hitting the light. I was in too big a hurry. Fortunately, before the nurse arrived, the little girl had a seizure. That was enough to persuade anyone. Her chemotherapy was stopped, and she was soon in the ICU. I'd gotten lucky, if luck it was.

The other time came when Brian, a boy of about eight who was newly diagnosed with leukemia, was getting his first dose of chemotherapy. Troubled by his declining awareness, I persuaded the resident to order a blood chemistry test. When that came back seriously out of kilter, the boy was rushed to the ICU, perhaps saving his life.

Notice how carefully I worked within the system. That was deliberate. I approached the staff closest to the patient to get changes made at the lowest possible level. Going higher only complicated matters. I also used arguments they understood and did my best to make the change seem reasonable. The bigger a change appeared, the more likely they'd pass it on to those higher up, creating a delay. Getting a boy's chemotherapy stopped on a mere hunch would have been hard. Getting a resident to order a test that would sound the alarm was better. Behind all of this, I tried to do my job well, so I'd be more believable in a crunch.

We'll look at the third problem in a couple of chapters. That's my search for a 'magic button' that would make the hospital take my hunches seriously no matter what.

Listen to Your Feelings

What I learned while caring for kids with leukemia applies equally well to situations where you need something changed, particularly situations involving suspicious guy behavior.

First, be everyone's favorite patient. Keep in mind what I said about the much-loved Binky. Make friends as soon as you arrive and before anything else happens. It's like having money in the bank. If trouble comes, you'll need to ask a lot of those caring for you. If they think you're special, it'll be much easier for them to take the heat for you.

Second, take your hunches seriously. They're often right, so don't let anyone put you down with, "Oh, you're just being a silly girl." But be careful. In most cases you shouldn't mention those feeling until you're ready to justify them with at least some specifics.

Third, see if your hunches have a sound foundation. Take a hard look at what you're feeling. If you don't like a staff guy simply because he looks like a guy at school you don't like, that doesn't count. Remember too that being weird is different from being creepy. A weird guy may have poor social skills, especially with girls, but he's likely to be harmless. He deserves pity more than fear.

A well-intentioned guy will be careful not to do things that leave you feeling uneasy. When I first began to work on the teen unit, I realized that I'd be around a lot of feminine undress, so I resolved to do everything I could to reassure those girls. I wouldn't hang around their room unnecessarily. I wouldn't contrive situations that'd expose them. I wouldn't look, however little they were wearing. A guy who means well does those sorts of things. He'll leave you feeling confident and in charge. You won't feel any more discomfort than necessary.

Fourth, it's suspicious behaviors that you're looking for. Look for things that make you feel uneasy. If he's a creep, they'll be there. A guy with a bad agenda may sound syrupy sweet, but behind his honeyed words, he will be pushing the limits of what he can get away with. You'll feel manipulated and controlled. That's because he doesn't care if you feel uneasy or if you find yourself pushed into embarrassing situations, as long as you go along. He wants you compliant, weak, and intimidated. He wants to be in control.

A Gift of Fear

If you have a chance, there's a book you might want to check out of a public library and look through. Although much of it is written for adults and people in business, *The Gift of Fear* by Gavin De Becker gives a wealth of helpful advice on how to sense risky guy-girl situations. When he writes for young women like you, he explains the warning signals, especially the gut-level feelings you should heed.

One chilling example he gives came on a flight from Chicago to Los Angeles. He was seated next to a teenaged girl traveling alone. Across the aisle was a man in his forties whose clothing suggested he'd just gotten out of prison.

That man started a conversation with the girl by saying "Hi, I'm Billy." The girl, no doubt wanting to be polite, gave her full name. Soon this Billy—if that was even his name—was pumping her for information, often using leading remarks: "I hate landing in a city and not knowing if anyone is meeting me." Foolishly, the girl responded by saying that she didn't know how she was getting from the airport to her destination, "The people I'm staying with are expecting me on a later flight." Bad, bad, bad.

Billy went on to suggest that, "you're probably not that independent." Being a teen, of course she had to reply that she was quite independent, having traveled on her own since thirteen. She didn't realize that she was being set up to show that independence by riding with him. He then insisted that she take a sip of his alcoholic drink, suggesting, "You sound like you play by your own rules." In a final move before going to the rest room, he leaned over and whispered to her, "Your eyes are awesome."

If you're feeling worried for this girl, you're getting the point both I and De Becker want to make. Here's how he summed up what had happened: "In a period of just a few minutes, I had watched Billy use forced teaming (they both had nobody meeting them, he said), too many details (the headphones and the woman he knows from Europe), loan sharking (the drink offer), charm (the compliment about the girl's eyes), and typecasting ('You're probably not that independent'). I had seen him discount the girl's 'no' when she declined the drink."

Notice Billy's aggressive familiarity and his attempt to find something in common with the girl. That's *forced teaming*, a way to "establish premature trust because we're in the same boat." *Too many details* is another warning, because those who deceive invent details to make their story seem more real. *Typecasting* is being critical in an effort to get you to react and move the other direction. *Loan sharking* is giving something (here a drink) to place you in their debt. De Becker goes on to warn you not to take promises seriously and to notice if a guy persists after you say 'no.' All these behaviors have the same goal—to take control away from you and put you in his power. The "gift of fear" of his title is the sense of unease you feel as this happens. Watch carefully for that feeling.

De Becker adds something else you may find helpful. "Remember, the nicest guy, the guy with no self-serving agenda whatsoever, the one who wants nothing from you, won't approach you at all."

That's an almost perfect description of what I did shortly before I worked at the hospital, when I spent four months traveling Europe by rail. In Southern Europe, I discovered that the pushy behavior of the local males toward young women from the U.S. left many of them eager to pair up with a guy like me for protection. Traveling alone most of the time, I was delighted to have their company.

Knowing that, did I approach these girls? No, I was careful to let them observe me and make the first move. I wanted to assure them that they were in control. They'd established our relationship. They could break it off whenever they chose. I wanted their companionship, but I wouldn't force it. No meant no.

A loss of control is what you should be watching for, even if he appears to be taking it away slowly, sweetly, and nicely. And it's often in the excesses where your danger signals lie—the sense that too much is going on. This guy is being too friendly. He seems too interested in you. He may offer too much help. Most important of all, he doesn't take 'no' for an answer. You may also get flashes of just how unkind he is if, for instance, he attempts to make you feel guilty for being suspicious.

Of course, the parallel between that plane flight and a hospital is far from perfect. In a hospital, guys on staff will always be approaching you. It's their job, so don't fault them for that. They also know your name and perhaps if you're lonely or vulnerable, so they don't need to question you about that. The fifteen-year-old Carina's sexually transmitted disease said all that a predator needed to know about her behavior, as we saw in the rapid inrush of those twisted male residents. But other factors can make a hospital particularly dangerous for you.

- You're sick and not in the best of shape for resisting a guy's moves.
- You're at a place where you're supposed to do what staff say, even when it involves exposure.
- The fact that the hospital is treating your illness and this guy is doing things for you can leave you feeling obligated.
- Being dependent on staff for your care can leave you feeling that you have no choice and must go along despite any discomfort you feel.

You'll notice that in this book I encourage you to resist those pressures. Don't let yourself be controlled or manipulated. If you sense that happening, stiffen your backbone, say no, and make it stick. The more someone pushes, the more strongly you should refuse, perhaps even breaking off all contact with a "leave my room now." Also, when you can, get support from others. Don't try to fight this alone.

In the chapters that follow, I'd be telling you how to act on those warning signs. To start with, I'll stress soft diplomatic responses to what even you're likely to agree are just unpleasant feelings and suspicions. That's because you're not going to be able to get other staff to respond aggressively to something vague. At best, this will win you a bit of distance from that guy and perhaps keep matters from moving on to something worse. That's usually enough.

Oh, and I imagine you'd like to hear what happened to that girl. When Billy left for the rest room, De Becker asked the girl if it was OK for him to talk with her. "It speaks to the power of the predatory strategies," he writes, "that she was glad to talk with Billy but a bit wary of a passenger (me) who asked permission to speak with her. 'He is going to offer you a ride from the airport,' I told her, "and he's not a good guy.'"

At baggage claim, De Becker saw Billy try to get her to ride with him. When she firmly said 'no,' the guy persisted, before finally walking away with an angry gesture that proved he wasn't the nice guy he'd pretended to be. All turned out well, and that girl learned a useful lesson. In the chapters that follow, I'll be offering you similar lessons adapted for a hospital.

29. Decide and Act

When I worked on the medical unit, our four-bed rooms mixed young boys and girls helter-skelter, because that made finding enough beds (or cribs) for them easier. That mixed bedding also explains the age when our young patients moved up to the teen unit, becoming 'teens' at a mere ten. "Why," I asked one hospital administrator, "do kids leave the medical unit at ten?" At the time, I thought something closer to puberty at twelve made more sense. Because, she told me, at about that age boys and girls develop a curiosity about each other that creates problems, minor though they be. Watching our kids, I decided she was right. When you're putting boys and girls in the same room, curiosity at ten is a better time for separate rooms than puberty at twelve.

That's the background to a problem that greeted me when I came to work one night while still working on the medical unit. But it wasn't childish curiosity that was the problem the evening nurse told us she'd just faced. Instead, it was the father of a little girl that, the nurse felt, was paying the wrong sort of attention to the other little girls in the room. That nurse acted on her 'something isn't quite right' feelings, much like I'm suggesting you do.

This evening nurse thought through carefully what she should do. Since parents didn't usually spend much time in those crowded four-bed rooms, she turned what was no more than general practice into a hard and fast rule and ordered that guy to leave. He left quietly and probably guiltily. If the nurse had done anything more official, perhaps accusing him and calling in security to evict him, things might have gotten messy.

Like that nurse, you may decide that your suspicions about a guy lurking and looking are real enough to need heeding. What should you do? Unfortunately, I can't give a simple answer. I'm going to make suggestions, and you'll have to pick what's best for your situation. Also, keep in mind that I'm assuming a generality, that you've got a nurse who is a woman and that the guy-creep who's bothering you is in some other staff position. If that's not the case, you'll need to make adjustments.

First, act quickly. As long what's happened is merely suspicious behavior, things like lurking and looking, you don't need to prove he's guilty in some absolute, court-of-law sense.

Remember, your goal at this point is to distance yourself from someone who makes you uncomfortable and not to get him officially branded as a pervert and fired. You're a patient and probably not feeling well. There's a lot you can't do. But you can act soon and while your discomfort is centered on look-see. The less you have to complain about—as long as it's something that matters—the more likely you are to be informally protected rather than forced into a nasty, bureaucratic battle over who is right. Take my word for it, you don't want to tangle with a hospital bureaucracy if you can avoid it.

Recall what I said about Jenny's must-have bath. All went well because she trusted me. But supposed a similar 'must do' situation came up with you, and your nurse gave the task to a guy who was making your skin crawl. If she already knows the guy makes you uncomfortable, she won't do that. Make sure she knows as soon as possible.

Second, don't worry about hurting a guy's feelings. Niceness has its limits. A good guy, one who's perhaps a bit clueless because he's new, will pick up what's happened and learn that there are things he shouldn't do—or at least not look like he is doing. That means you'll actually be doing him a favor. On the other hand, a creep won't care how you feel, so there's no need to fret about his feelings. Go ahead and criticize him with my blessings.

Third, decide who'll talk. If you have no trouble speaking your mind, then by all means take care of it yourself. You're the witness and the one most affected. That counts for a lot. It also keeps what you say more casual than if your parents do the talking.

If you're shy and unassertive, don't let that keep you from acting. As I wrote earlier, before you come to the hospital have someone set up to speak for you about troubles from bad food to creepy guys. That might be your dad or mom, because the hospital knows they have legal rights. It might be an aunt, uncle, or family friend who's a doctor or nurse. Being in medicine creates a common ground with staff. Or it might be a brother, sister, or friend who has no problem being assertive. The important thing is to have someone who is persuasive on your side. You shouldn't have to fight this alone. You're the one who's sick.

Fourth, decide who to talk with. In most cases, a nurse you like and trust is the best choice, particularly if she's on duty when the problem happens. She's in charge of your moment-to-moment care, and for that her word is law. Win her to your side, and she can take care of those who are under her, perhaps along with auxiliary staff, such as physical therapists and medical technicians, should the creep be one of those. Go any higher than her, say to the head nurse, and you've moved into administration. That means policies, formality and paperwork, exactly what you want to avoid at this point.

That said, if you're not close to the nurse who's on duty when the creep is around, consider someone who's more sympathetic—perhaps a nursing assistant. People who work together day after day often develop a trust and an attitude of mutual aid. I could get the nurses I worked with to do something simply as a favor to me. If that's what it takes to get your problem solved, go for it.

Remember too what I said about some guys being more sensitive to guy-see-girl issues than women. You may find the best person to approach is the right guy, one who'll be happy to help you—a blushing damsel in distress. Persuade him, and your problem is over. He's more likely to understand a creep and less likely to play feminine 'smiles and niceness.' If necessary, he might even take the creep aside and tell him, "Hey, you're bothering her. I like her. Stay away." A direct approach like that can work wonders. Most creeps are cowards—that's why they prey on young women. And there's no way he can protest that guy's warning without drawing attention to himself. That he doesn't want to do.

Fifth, make the talk informal and off the record. That's easiest if you're doing the talking. Ask the nurse (or whoever) for a few minutes and make it alone if possible. If you're in a room with other girls and can't get out of bed, you might even whisper in one another's ears, creating a nice 'conspiratorial' feeling that may make the nurse more sympathetic. The fewer who hear, the better.

If someone else is speaking for you, keeping that informality is a bit harder. Talking face to face means coming down to the hospital. If possible, contrive a normal visit from your mom and then have her tell your nurse, "Oh, could I talk to you a minute about my daughter? She really thinks you're a great nurse, and we need your help with something." That lets the nurse know she's not the problem. Remember that the nurse is likely to busy (particularly at hours divisible by four and near shift change), so arrange a time when she's free.

If coming down to the hospital is hard, given distance, traffic, and work schedules, consider telling the nurse, "Oh, I've told my dad what a great nurse you are, and he wants to talk with you about something. When you've got a couple of minutes free, I'll get him on my cell phone." Talking on your phone (when possible) not only lets the nurse go somewhere private, initiating it yourself makes it a little less official. Remember, at this point you want results rather than a confrontation.

In what follows, I assume you'll be talking to your nurse about an assistant. Keep in mind it might be someone else, including a male nurse, a resident physician, or even one of the hospital's senior physicians.

Sixth, strike a careful balance between frivolous and serious. Enter the conversation knowing you'll be walking a tightrope that demands your best people skills. Make the situation seem too slight, and nothing will change. Make it seem too serious, and the nurse will feel she has to tell those over her. When you talk, keep your focus on your feelings, stressing that they are reasonable feelings, and suggest a simple way they can be made better. The same is true if your mother or father are talking. Either can stress that "this has our daughter upset and uncomfortable." They don't need to prove a crime to get those unpleasant circumstances changed and your feelings improved.

That means you should bring in enough evidence to show that you're not a silly girl with an overactive imagination. But keep in mind that, past a certain point, the nurse may decide that the evidence requires her to report what you're saying. That could turn into a terrible 'he said, she said' situation with the hospital, prodded by its lawyer, likely to take the guy's side. That's why it's best to act when the problem is small—things like looking rather than touching or groping.

Saying That Again

It's important, so I'll say it again. At this stage, focus on the discomfort this guy is causing you rather than on proving a serious offense. In most hospitals, nurses have a lot of discretionary power. On her own, a nurse can act on your feelings and make adjustments in your care just to make you feel more comfortable. That's part of being a nurse. She doesn't have to prove you're right to make those changes.

And no, that doesn't mean this creep gets off scot-free. Nurses are chatty about their patients and other staff. If other girls make similar complaints, something will eventually be done, but it'll be done by several nurses acting in concert. Hospital politics can be brutal. Better them than you.

So keep your goals modest. The less you're asking for, as long as it's enough to make you feel OK, the easier it'll be for a nurse to help you on her own. If bedpans, baths, and linen changes are what leave you uncomfortable, she can handle the first and perhaps get a nearby female nursing assistant to handle the other two. If more than that is needed, in a pinch a helpful nurse can take over all your care, moving the creep out of all contact with you. If she's the nurse and he's an assistant, she doesn't have to give a reason.

When the problem can't fixed, you may have to come up with solutions that depend totally on you. If he is lurking and looking, be careful to stay covered up when he's around. Don't be afraid to be obvious either. Glaring at him is perfectly OK, and coldly ignoring his existence is probably even better. If you're in a room with other girls, tell them too. Make him uncomfortable. That should keep him away.

Finally, at this stage do your best to keep what's happening unofficial. If you push matters up one level, typically to the head nurse, all of a sudden what you've been feeling has become an accusation and what you're saying has become an incident. In most cases, the head nurse will have to file a report, and a formal investigation will follow. Then things will get emotionally intense and draining. Better to win a little victory and get peace of mind than face a big hassle and the chance of losing.

That seeming informality doesn't mean that you should not be documenting what's happening in a diary or with a cell phone. Like I said earlier, if matters turn serious and legal, other witnesses, notes, and time-stamped text messages will be important. Don't see that as a hassle. See it as an adventure. Turn your hospital stay into a story.

Next, I'll deal with how to handle situations where either nothing has been done despite your efforts to keep it low-key, or where something has happened that must be formally deal with. Either is a situation where any trouble you may cause is less important than getting results.

30. MAGIC BUTTONS

It's late at night and that thin hospital gown that's all you're wearing is blowing in the cold wind, leaving you chilled to the bone. Your feet are growing numb, because the little paper slip-ons you're wearing offer no protection. Even worse, you're waiting at a bus stop near the hospital, and you keep glancing over your shoulder in horror at two spooky looking guys who've been eyeing you from about ten feet away. "If only that bus would come," you keep thinking, "and if only I hadn't been so insistent at the hospital, I wouldn't be here."

Now banish that thought completely and utterly from your mind. You're not going to be tossed out of a hospital for doing anything I suggest in this book. If anything, the hospital staff will respect you all the more. Just remember what I've said about being appreciative and helpful from the moment you arrive, as well as being sensitive to the many pressures hospital staff operate under. Treat them with kindness and respect, and they will treat you the same. You don't have to be the Queen of All Ill-Tempered Patients to get the care you deserve. Sweetness and firmness can accomplish a lot.

In fact, what that terrible scene at a bus stop describes is known as patient abandonment, and it's a serious violation of medical ethics, one fraught with severe legal penalties. In 2007, one California court ruled that, "abandonment of a case by a physician without sufficient notice or adequate excuse is a dereliction of duty, and if injury results there from, the physician may be held liable in damages." So no hospital that's worth staying at is going to stop treatment or toss you out for insisting on not being embarrassed. That would be most unprofessional.

OK, now we need to move on to the really hard problems, nasty situations that there's a slight possibility—and only a slight one—that you might face during your stay in a hospital. Throughout this book, I've been encouraging you to be assertive and take charge of the parts of your medical care that matter to you, particularly things that embarrass you or make you feel uncomfortable. At the same time, I've stressed the importance of being appreciative, kind and understanding of those taking care of you. All that is good, but that may not be enough.

Pushing Magic Buttons

Now, I'm going to deal with situations where you may need to be assertive enough that you upset those at the hospital, perhaps even your new hospital friends. That's all right. In most cases, that's because your efforts to solve a problem informally have failed or because something serious has happened. Earlier, I talked about Binky and a 'magic tip' to get hospital staff to look out for you. That still applies. But now I'm going to talk about a 'magic button' to force matters to go your way.

What do I mean by a magic button? In much of life, there are words someone can say to force a system to take them seriously, typically to protect people from great harm or death. An airplane pilot in trouble can declare an emergency and demand that air traffic controllers land him immediately at the nearest airfield, even if the resulting confusion leaves air traffic over the city in a mess for hours.

U.S. Coast Guard officers have similar power. I saw a documentary in which someone caught in a terrible storm radioed for a helicopter to come far offshore to take off his passenger but wanted to stay with his sailboat. Given the severity of the storm, in a few hours the boat owner might be calling for another rescue flight, putting a helicopter crew again at risk, so a Coast Guard officer formally declared the sailboat 'manifestly unsafe.' If the owner refused to leave after that declaration, he could be prosecuted, and his boat impounded. He complied.

In short, magic buttons are good things. They make people do what needs to be done. They do, however, need to be used carefully.

A Nurse's Magic Button

Nurses at the hospital where I worked had a magic button. A nurse who disagreed with the treatment being given one of her patients could object and a fast-moving formal process would begin—even if she was a new nurse only a few weeks out of nursing school.

Whatever the time, day or night, when she objected to a medical order, the attending physician—the one specifically responsible for that patient's care—had to be contacted and required to approve or disapprove the treatment yet again. What followed became his responsibility in a much more serious sense. If the treatment still stood, the nurse could insist that either the chief of medicine or chief of surgery for the entire hospital be called, with perhaps the hospital's CEO also involved. Matters then got very dicey. It meant that the hospital itself became responsible in a most serious way if something went wrong. It could no longer plead "But we didn't know." What had been routine was now fraught with consequences, medical, ethical and legal. That magic button gave a young, inexperienced but brave nurse enormous power. She would be heard. That was good.

My Magic Button

Earlier, I mentioned the hunches I had that a patient was in trouble—hunches that were never wrong. In three cases when I got that feeling, the child was in the ICU within hours. In the fourth, a little girl was rushed to emergency surgery. That brings up the third problem those hunches created for me—one I wrestled with almost my entire time at the hospital. What if I became convinced that one of my children was in serious trouble and that her treatment had to be changed, but I was unable to persuade either my nurse or the resident on duty? It was the middle of the night. There was no one more important around. What could I do? In a matter of minutes, that child might be dead. I didn't want to be proved right after the fact. I wanted the child to live. But as an aide, I didn't have that nurse's magic button.

What I needed was a never-fail way to get a child the attention she needed. I had to make sure phone calls would go out, day or night, awakening a child's attending physician, a nationally ranked expert whose judgment I respected. And, whatever happened to the alarm I'd raised, I needed to make sure that everyone would be watching that child like a hawk for the next few critical hours. If what I did put my job on the line, then so be it. I could always find another job. That child could not find another life. In *Nights with Leukemia*, I describe how I found that magic button during my last few weeks at the hospital. What I found was a most dangerous button, but it would have the desired effect.

We'll now look at the magic buttons that are available to you as a patient. Whether you should use them and which you should use depends on your situation. Just be careful. Some can be risky.

31. Making "No" Stick

Remember Carina, the pretty fifteen-year-old who couldn't say no and endured at least eight highly intrusive pelvic exams in a matter of minutes before being rescued by her nurse? That's what we'll be talking about here—serious situations that have gone beyond lingering looks and your need to get distance from someone who simply makes you feel uncomfortable. Here we'll be talking about situations that you either don't want to happen at all, or that you want to stop immediately. This is about saying "No" and making it stick.

Dealing with Trouble

Keep in mind that your situation doesn't have to be as bad as Carina's to qualify for immediate action. What matters is that you are finding yourself overwhelmed by unwanted attention and perhaps getting 'inspected' in places or ways that make you feel uncomfortable. The circumstances may be suspicious—too many eager young males lurking about being the most obvious. As with Carina, it may involve examinations being repeated over and over again, making it obvious this isn't about helping you. Then again, it may just involve one person, but happening in ways you find suspicious or creepy.

The key issue here is professionalism. When I worked in a hospital, I always saw myself as responsible for whatever went wrong. I should have prepared better. I should have explained better—that sort of thing. That was particularly true with dying children. The family was facing a child's death for the first time and under a lot of stress. Their mistakes and emotions were understandable and excusable. In contrast, I did that all the time. I should know how to do it right. Whatever went wrong was my mistake, so I was the one who must learn and change. That's what being a professional means. A professional is always responsible.

The same is true with how staff handle your feelings of discomfort. Those treating you should behave like professionals. Remember, you're not a chunk of meat to be flipped about on a grill. No matter how serious your illness, it's not your responsibility to grit your teeth and endure what happens. It's the responsibility of staff to talk with you, explain what'll be done, and make you comfortable.

Perhaps the best principle to keep in mind is that it's better to avoid a problem than to deal with it in a crisis. Don't hesitate to make it clear from the start of your hospital stay that you're not an 'anything goes' or 'can't say no' sort of girl. Whether you're easily embarrassed like Min or simply have a set of firm 'what guys can do' rules like Nina, Heidi, and the Twins, make sure that's widely known. In most cases, the staff will make adjustments without you having to do anything more.

In addition, if your attitudes are based on your religious beliefs, don't hesitate to make that known. Unlike Europe, where state churches were and still are the norm, this country was founded to offer religious freedom for all. There are numerous laws and court decisions that back up medical choices based on religious faith. Hospitals know that. Doctors and nurses have been taught to respect religious views. If that's true in your case, don't hesitate to make that known. That will help. If you're at a loss for words, tell them that your religion is "like the Amish," and they'll find you fascinating.

Be diplomatic. When you bring up a problem, you might frame it as a question and let the staff find the best answer. That uses their expertise and makes you seem less bossy. In Min's case, she might have said, "I embarrass very easily. How can I make sure that I don't get uncovered when someone turns me over?" Most nurses are smart and caring people. True, they are busy and may be inclined to view teen-girl undress casually. But if they know how you feel, they can adjust how you're cared for. In most cases, if you tell one nurse, she'll tell the others. Nurses like to pass along that sort of thing.

OK, so you're bothered, upset or even creeped out and ready to make that known. What should you do? I've talked about magic buttons. What are yours?

1. Withholding Consent

Consent is your most powerful button because it's based on law. Medical care requires your permission or, if you're not quite of age, that of your parents. The fact that examinations and treatment require your consent means you can say no and make it stick. When you don't like something, make it clear as firmly and politely as you can that you're not giving your permission. The paperwork that you or your parents signed when you came to the hospital does give them a general right to treat you, but that doesn't mean that you can't alter the specifics.

Yes, in emergency, there is something called implied consent that covers situations where you are unconscious and bleeding badly. But if you're alert and lying in a hospital bed looking up, the simple fact that you're sick doesn't give doctors the right to treat you anyway they want.

It's also true that you can, in certain situations, even refuse life-saving treatment. But that's not what we're talking about here.

Keep in mind that hospital staff, particularly the doctors, aren't used to hearing "no." They're used to giving orders and being obeyed. With that in mind, do your best not to stand alone. That's why I stress making friends on staff as soon as you arrive. A nurse can disagree with a doctor and win. I've seen that happen.

Also, many people find the first point of view they hear the most believable. If your parents need to be involved, do your best let them know in advance and, if a crisis develops, be the first to inform them. Make the call yourself and hang on to the phone come what may. (If necessary, use both hands.) Before you talk with them, take a deep breath, then speak calmly and clearly about what's happening. Hysterics are not a good idea. The better you explain, the better your chances of success, and the less likely you'll feel railroaded, even if they agree with your doctor.

2. Yes, But Only If

Your second button, one you'll probably want to use much more often than a flat no, might be called "Yes, but only if." In this case, you set conditions under which you will accept this procedure. You're telling them, "If you do this, I'll let you do that."

For instance, who's present for a procedure may matter to you. I always left an exam room or a bedside the instant I realized that something was about to happen where my presence wasn't required and that might embarrass a girl. Not all guys do that though, so if it's a guy or clique of guys hanging around that bother you, simply say: "Sorry, I hate to make trouble, but I'll only agree to this if these guys leave." If the guys don't like that, tough. Remember, you're a patient and not a mannequin in a store window, to be dressed and undressed at will.

If someone says they need to look on to learn, again that's tough for them. They can learn on a teen guy or a more willing girl. They can even try procedures on themselves. Some nurses I worked with practiced starting IVs on one another. That teaches how patients feel.

3. First, Talk with Me

The third button might be called, "First, talk to me." With it, you insist on getting information and being satisfied with what you hear before agreeing or not. Here, you're asking for an explanation why this procedure is necessary, as well as details about who and what is involved.

It's what they should be doing anyway, so you're helping them do their job. Several factors might matter to you.

First, there's the yuck factor. Getting a needle stuck into your backbone isn't pleasant to think about. Pala, overwhelmed as she was, had a right to know that the procedure was necessary, that it wasn't just part of some obscure research protocol. Before her chemotherapy started—and that needed to be soon—we had to look at her spinal fluid to see if leukemia cells had spread there. That could affect her treatment. She had a right to know that. She (meaning you) shouldn't be bounced from procedure to procedure without a word of explanation.

Yes, given Pala's dreadful situation, it was hard for her to insist on being told. But you may be in a stronger position than she was, if for no more reason than that you've read this most inspiring book. If you insist on an explanation, even when it's not strictly necessary, you establish a pattern that will also apply to girls such as Pala. By insisting on an answer, you help girls like her and remind a hospital what it ought to do.

Second, there's the embarrassment factor. That lumbar puncture was emotionally as well as physically intrusive. The back of Pala's gown was open, the resident was bending close and poking her in the small of her back. I had her pinned down so she couldn't move. I did my best, using a towel as a surgical drape, but it wasn't perfect. If I hadn't done that, she'd have been within her rights to ask to be better covered. So don't be ashamed to insist on changes simply because they make you feel better. Many in medicine need better manners, particularly in-training residents. You do them a favor by insisting that they act better.

The third might be called the "who's there" factor. In the case of Pala, it happened that we were both guys. As a girl, should you be flexible about that or insist on all or mostly women to do intrusive things?

Your comfort level is a good guide. Ask yourself "Is this something I can accept and forget, or is this something that'll still bother me long after I go home?" A poke in the small of your back isn't as embarrassing as a lengthy vaginal exam. For the former, a guy resident may be tolerable, assuming he knows what he is doing. For the latter, feel free to insist on having a woman or at least a much older male doctor. Never forget that the choice is yours. If it really matters to you, don't be afraid to say, "It's my way or the highway."

The number of people present is a fourth factor. Ask in advance or look around and see how many people are in the room. Most non-surgical procedures require only two or at the most three people, since that's about all that can get around you comfortably. If that matters to you, it's fine to not want lookers-on. If more than are needed are present, feel free to ask the rest to leave.

Like I said, that isn't the end of the world for the hospital. Most patients go along with almost anything. They can learn on them rather than you. But remember, if it's not that big a deal with you, it helps to be flexible. Establish that you are in charge from the start, so they respect you and defer to your wishes. But do your best to save those protests and refusals for what really matters. Fighting everything is likely to leave you too tired to fight over what really matters.

Competence is the fifth factor and matters the most. Remember Pala's badly botched spinal tap. You have a right to know that those doing a procedure know what they're doing. After all you're the one who's going to be poked, prodded or inspected.

Here you're in a unique position of power. You can do things I couldn't do as a member of the hospital staff. I knew nothing about the resident who was doing Pala's spinal tap. That day was the first time I'd seen him. If I'd tried to question his competence—as opposed to concluding afterward that he was a dolt—I'd have gotten into big trouble. He outranked me in the hospital hierarchy, so I might have been told that I had no right to question his skills, all the more loudly if he doubted those skills himself. Even more important, someone senior to him had sent him, so by questioning that resident's competence, I'd also be questioning their judgment. The result might have been a minor fire storm. Hospital politics is nasty.

But you're not part of that hospital hierarchy. You have every right to question someone's skills. But how do you know if you should? After all, you're not a doctor or a nurse. Well, you don't need to have a medical degree to make a judgment call. Look at how well he explains the procedure to you—assuming he even does that. (If not, insist on it.) And when he starts, see if he moves smoothly, quickly and confidently, perhaps while talking calmly with you. Does he fumble with instruments, or handle them with skill? Does he seem to be struggling with what to do next or to know instinctively. All those indicate if he knows what he is doing.

If the person about to do the procedure seems clumsy or uncertain, speak up. Remind yourself that what you want is reasonable—competent, capable care. Ask the resident or doctor how many times he has done the procedure before, and, if you get a vague answer or a low number, feel free to be firm and say, "Well, you need to either get someone else to do the procedure or at least find someone more experienced to supervise you. I'll be happy to wait here in the exam room while you get them." That's saying no, but offering a way out. Remember, there are more important things in life that not irritating someone who's likely to forget your name in an hour or two anyway. He'll get over it.

Most important of all, keep in mind that you don't need to know everything to be safe. You can tap into the knowledge of those caring for you. That's what happened when Carina's nurse heard what was going on in the exam room and intervened. That's why I put so much stress on becoming someone the staff like, so they 'go the extra mile' for you. When you don't know much, it helps to have people around who do and who like you. They can intervene or back you up when you protest.

Remember your right to ask about and even refuse a part of your medical care based on the reasons I've described above. That's your most important magic button. And if someone gives you a hard time about that, particularly if they make threats, make it clear that if they continue to harass you, you will file a formal complaint. Verbal abuse and bullying are most unprofessional and never acceptable in a hospital. Politely insist on being treated with respect. Keep your cool and force them keep theirs. In most disagreements, the one who stays calm wins.

4. A Real Doctor

There's a fourth magic button that some find quite effective in both clinics and hospitals, particularly when they're getting stupid, intrusive or substandard care from inexperienced doctors and residents. Call it the "real doctor" button. Legally, it carries little weight. If they have MD after their name, they're a real doctor under the law. But emotionally, the term is powerful because it links being new to medicine with being unskilled. Just use it with care. It can really tick people off. The newer they are to medicine, the less happy they'll be with being told that they're not a real doctor.

How do you use this button? You push it by insisting that you be treated by a "real doctor" and repeating that over and over again, refusing to be draw into medical criteria you know nothing about. Since the hospital itself recognizes that residents aren't quite real doctors and that even some of those who've finished their residency are still learning, what you're saying carries a great deal of emotional weight. Hospitals know that some physicians are more capable than others, so you're applying their own standards to them. You're insisting on getting someone better. That's only fair. After all, it's you who'll suffer the consequences of a blunder.

You might take matters one step further by defining what you mean by a real doctor. "I want to be examined by one doctor only, and I want that doctor to be experienced in this procedure and at least 35 years old." If it makes you feel better, add, "And I want this exam to be done by a woman." If privacy is your chief concern, you might relent a bit on the age and experience to settle for a woman. Just keep in mind that staffing limitations may mean that not all your conditions are doable. But what you're demanding should stop an uncomfortable situation in its tracks and get at least some changes made. Remember, making a stand once is likely to get you treated better on other occasions without you having to do anything more. Hospitals hate 'scenes.'

Next, we'll look at much messier situations where saying no comes too late to keep you from being hurt. Something has happened that you need to formally protest—something most unpleasant. I hope that never happens to you, but it may, and it helps to be prepared.

32. Going Nuclear

The letter was my parting gift for the hard-working teen nurses that I'd been with for some ten months. I liked every one of them and wanted to ease their grim workload. In my resignation from the hospital, I asked the head of nursing to make several changes on the teen unit, the most important being to shift as much work as possible from an overworked day shift to an underworked evening shift. If the hospital's head of nursing took those complaints as my reason for leaving, so much the better. I was actually leaving for graduate study in medical ethics—what I called "studying law in the medical school." But being overloaded with busy work on teen day shift was one reason why I wasn't interested in turning my full-time day position, a prized possession in any hospital, into a student-friendly weekend-days-only one. School would be more than enough to keep me busy.

Putting It On Paper

By making my criticism in a letter, I turned my suggestions into a formal complaint, which is what we'll talk about in this chapter. I didn't discuss my criticism with the nurses I was working with, because they already understood the problem but were poorly placed to do anything about it. Some might accuse them of shirking if they'd raised the issues. I was leaving, so those accusations didn't bother me.

Nor did I take my complaints informally to the unit's head nurse. That was pointless, because her mind was closed. She'd returned from maternity leave a few months before and, without bothering to investigate, immediately attacked our overworked nurses for doing a poor job. With me, she'd become threatening, claiming that the unit was going to have fewer aides and hoping I'd try to make myself look better by finding fault with my nurses. Since I felt all were doing good work, I refused. To this day I remain proud of that.

The head nurse was not happy when she heard about my letter to her boss and told me so when we met for the last time. I didn't care. I'd made my point, and the impact was already being felt. Two of my three complaints had come up at a staff meeting a few days after I turned in my letter. Like it or not, the hospital was having to act. I'd done what I could. I'd put my complaints in writing.

Making a Formal Complaint

You may face something similar while you're in a hospital. It may center on something that you've been unable to get dealt with by the more informal methods I've described thus far, or it may be an incident so awful, you can't let it pass. Finally, it could be a hospital practice or policy that you believe needs to be changed, so other patients don't get hurt like you did. Whatever it is, you want the hospital to act and don't mind stirring up some dust along the way.

Yes, I know. In this book, I've done my best to help you avoid formal complaints. I've described how to get staff on your side and sympathetic. I encouraged you to take charge of your care and deal with issues while they're still small. I've described informal ways to get problems fixed. Most of the time, that should be enough.

But as with me and that overwork, you could find yourself in a situation where nothing informal works. You must either give up doing anything or make a formal complaint. Formal as in paperwork. Formal as in evidence-gathering, hearings, policies, procedures, and committees. Not my cup of tea and probably not yours either. But if you want action, that's what you may have to do. You have to 'go nuclear.'

What does making a formal complaint involve? Obviously, that depends on your hospital. I'd suggest that you start by either approaching or having your parents approach the hospital administration, asking how to make a complaint.

That's likely to mean that the hospital will try to talk you out of making that formal complaint by solving the problem to your satisfaction. If that happens, take full advantage of it. They want to please you, so let them. If you can solve your problem that way, go for it. If not, be aware that making a formal complaint may shift them from being helpful to being defensive. It could get tense.

I'll add something else you should know. If your complaint is the sort that legal systems take seriously, you're more likely to find the hospital cooperative because they know you can take them to court. If they were supposed to amputate your right leg and they took off your left leg instead ("Yikes!"), they know they're in big trouble and must settle as soon as possible.

Unfortunately, embarrassment issues and even more serious issues such as groping, aren't as clear-cut legally as they should be. A court is likely to say, 'So what, this is a hospital' to any claim you make about embarrassment, and charges of groping can quickly turn into a nasty 'he said, she said' dispute that gets nowhere and may leave you screaming in frustration.

Doing Research

I saw that lack of interest in embarrassment issues when I sat down with a research librarian at the best-equipped medical library in my state. She and I spent the better part of an hour looking through online databases for medical articles on patient embarrassment at any age and not just for teen girls. We drew a complete blank.

I spent another hour looking through dozens of nursing guidebooks, again drawing a blank. As I write this, patient embarrassment, much less that of sensitive teen girls, doesn't seem to be a major issue within either medicine or nursing. That's one reason why I'm writing this, and why I hope you and I break new ground. Something must be done.

What that librarian and I did find was one article that debated the merits of having a second person in the room for intimate exams, just in case the patient goes to court with some charge. It concluded that, unless the legal situation changed, that wasn't necessary. That's bad news for you, because that says that, at present in a 'he said, she said' dispute in court, he is likely to win under 'beyond a shadow of a doubt' reasoning. Since hospitals are unlikely to lose in court, the article concluded, there's no need for them to make policies that require at least two staff to be present for intimate exams. Keep in mind that's for something serious, such as charges of groping, and not just a staff guy lurking about your room behaving like a creep. Sadly, the law isn't weighed in your favor. It's unlikely to be your friend.

Moving On

If you can't always use a threat of going to court to light a fire under a hospital administration, what can you do? That all depends on just how good—in the caring about people sense—that hospital is. You can discover that by watching hospital staff at work.

Do they seem happy with what they're doing? If so, the hospital is treating them well and is likely to treat you the same. Good morale is a sign of good leadership. Does the staff seem eager to provide you with good care? If so, then the hospital is likely to take your complaint seriously. You're in a good hospital.

On the other hand, if the staff seem discouraged and indifferent, your best option might not be a formal complaint, since that's likely to prove a waste of time. It may be to transfer to a different hospital, something your doctor should be able to arrange. Be glad that you can still do that. Not everyone can.

When I did a Google search a few days ago for "hospital formal complaint," there were over 12 million results. That's a depressingly large number. Great Britain is clearly where you don't want to be sick. Four of the top five hits were for the hospitals there. In fact the Britain's National Health Service (NHS) "Complaints" web page was Google's top hit. Read it and weep for those tea-sippers across the Atlantic. Here's what is said under "What are my rights?"

The NHS Constitution explains your rights when it comes to making a complaint. You have the right to:

- *Have your complaint dealt with efficiently, and properly investigated,*
- *Know the outcome of any investigation into your complaint,*
- *Take your complaint to the independent Parliamentary and Health Service Ombudsman if you're not satisfied with the way the NHS has dealt with your complaint,*
- *Make a claim for judicial review if you think you've been directly affected by an unlawful act or decision of an NHS body, and*
- *Receive compensation if you've been harmed.*

Limited Choices

Do you see what's missing? There's no "right to take your health care elsewhere." Yes, the web page has "NHS Choices" at the top and that's literally true. Your only choices are those the NHS offers. They're not your choices. They're their choices. They chose if you get treated, as well as when and how. They chose what hospital you use, and what tests are run. They even choose who cares for you, including that guy who makes your skin crawl. You can like it or lump it. What you can't do, unless your parents are well-off, is leave it.

If you choose to complain, you must do it the NHS way. It's all stiff, formal and bureaucratic, with investigators, ombudsman, and judicial review. The system is policing the system. A hospital knows how to work that system. It has people whose full time job is doing just that. If you were a patient there, you'd find the mechanics of complaining confusing, particularly while you're battling a major illness. That's because, although you can complain, your complaints have no teeth. You have no real alternative. And yes, if you have enough money, you can have your health care handled privately. But that rewards rather than punishes the NHS. If you go private, the NHS no longer has to cover the cost of your care. Flip the coin as many times as you want, it always comes up the same. Heads they win. Tails you lose.

Here in the United States, you've got far more leverage (at least for now), because hospitals have to compete for your care and bad hospitals suffer the consequences. If you bring your parents' health care insurance with you, you're in particularly good shape because you're the one who's paying. That makes you the fiddler calling the tune. Unlike the NHS, if you walk, they lose. Among administrators that matters a lot, and it's they who'll be handling your formal complaint.

So, realize that your ability to chose who does your care gains you leverage. You can threaten to leave if changes aren't made.

Gaining More Leverage

Not leaving quietly gives you still more leverage, although it should be used only as a last resort. It can make you some powerful enemies.

Hospitals fear bad publicity, especially in the local news media. They are afraid that patients will hear about what happened to you and go elsewhere. They worry that doctors will refer patients to another hospital. They fret that bad press means their hospital rankings will be lowered. They even fear wealthy donors may give to some other charity. Fear is not the best of motivators, but it does get results.

I once heard a mother speak about what happened when she went to enroll her teen daughter in a public school system for the first time. Her daughter had Downs syndrome and had been educated at home. But now that she was older, the mother felt she would benefit from being in a school with a broader social life.

Unfortunately, when she went to arrange that, the school officials told her that the school would not guarantee that her daughter would be safe from sexual assault, and that they required that she place her daughter on birth control pills, as if pregnancy were the only issue.

The mother, as you might expect, went ballistic and told us how she dealt with those bureaucrats. "I have friends who work for local television news teams," she told them. "You will either do whatever it takes to protect my daughter, or I will go to them with this story. Do you really want the lead story on the evening news to be your refusal to protect my daughter from being raped?" Faced with that ultimatum, the school relented. There's power in publicity.

Do you or your parents have those connections? If so and if the situation justifies taking that action, then you may want to be prepared to do so. If not, then be prepared to face the fact that, once you've made a formal complaint, matters are out of your hands. With the informal methods I've described, you can charm the staff, persuading them to help you. You can pick the nurse you talk with, perhaps choosing the kindest. When you're dealing with a bureaucracy, none of that is in your hands. Decisions you consider important will be made by people you've never met. That can be frustrating.

Finally, if all else fails, the state in which you live will have an agency that regulates hospitals, typically as part of a department of health. You can file a formal complaint with them. You may or may not be successful there, but at least you'll be on record as filing a complaint.

And yes, I'm most sorry for all this glumness about formal complaints. I know that when you're sick enough to be hospitalized, the last thing you want is get into a drawn-out battle with strangers. Sometimes the fight just isn't worth the trouble. But I did not want to leave that option out. In some cases it may work, particularly if you have a case that's well supported by evidence. If nothing else, your complaint will be added to others and may eventually bring changes.

We'll wrap up by looking at what we've learned.

33. Miss Buns and the Wet Hens

On the teen unit, the first half-hour in the morning was always the busiest. I'd check the vital signs (temperature etc.) for my ten or more patients and then, when the breakfast trays arrived, deliver one to each bed. Breakfast in bed was one of the few luxuries we offered our unfortunate captives. Get behind then, and my whole day would be a mess.

Usually, I'd check first the multi-bed room that seemed most awake. This day, it was the boys room. A few minutes later, when I entered the girls room, I knew something was amiss. Three of the girls—girls I'd never had as patients before—were glaring at me like wet hens. The fourth girl was why. Despite the bright morning sun pouring in the windows, she was lying on her tummy, pretending to sleep. The back of her gown was open, showing her girlish buns. She'd come in the evening before, probably slept that way at home, and saw no reason to change in a hospital.

I knew the three angry Wet Hens wanted me to leave post-haste, but I couldn't do that. I had too little time as is. If they'd been that concerned, I told myself, one of them could have gotten out of bed, covered her up, and whispered something girlish in her ear. The night nurse, I also lamented, could have taken care of this.

Normally, I'd have just gone over and covered Miss Buns up. But with the three Wet Hens glaring at me, I knew that'd only change my status in their eyes from "Peeping Tom" to "Peeping Tom Goes Closer." I didn't want that. Instead, I avoided looking at Miss Buns and skipped her vital signs. That I had the time to do later.

A few minutes later, when I delivered the breakfast trays, I was happy to find Miss Buns sitting up, all prim and proper. The nurses were relaxed about what girls wore in their room. It was, after all, their room. But they were strict about what the boys next door could see, and Miss Buns was visible from the doorway. Eventually, the Wet Hens unruffled their feathers and decided I wasn't quite as bad as they'd first thought.

The Wet Hens experience came near the end of my time at the hospital. That's why I had that "I can only do so much" response to their girlish outrage. As a guy, I'd come to accept that there were limits to how well I could deal with undressed teen girls. There was simply no way I could please everyone across a gap as wide as that between the angry Wet Hens and little Miss Buns.

Divided Memories

Odd as it may sound, when I left the hospital about a month later, a split opened up in my memory about my experiences. I thought often about my time in Hem-Onc, but I almost never recalled those teen-girl frustrations. The first, thanks to all the expertise at caring for the dying that had surrounded me, was fulfilling. The second, in an environment where even mentioning the word embarrassment seemed forbidden by some unspoken rule, left me feeling that much had been left unresolved. What I had learned, I learned through trial and error, hating my mistakes, but appreciating the kindness these girls had shown me.

That selective remembering is why, as I began writing the companion to this book, *Nights with Leukemia*, I didn't know I'd also be writing this one. I was surprised when the memories you've been reading here began to surface in my mind. It was like what happened to J. R. R. Tolkien as he wrote *The Lord of the Rings*. As he created the draft, he was amazed to discover new characters appearing unbidden as he pecked away at his typewriter. Who is this guy, he would ask, and what part does he play in my story? Like him, I was surprised to find these real people and their experiences reappearing in my thoughts.

Memories Return

The entering wedge was Carina. How she was treated, particularly by those residents, so angered me that I'd never forgotten her. I felt her story needed to come out—as indeed it will in a third (and free digital) book called *Carina, The Girl Who Couldn't Say No*. As I thought about what happened to her, my other experiences with these teen girls came back into my conscious mind, unbidden and unexpected. I soon realized I had another book in the making.

Two things surprised me about those returning memories. The first was their clarity after so long. Most memories fade if we don't regularly remind ourselves of them. These were as clear as if they'd happened the day before. The second was that, as I began to fit these memories into a book, I discovered that they already formed a coherent story. I have only one explanation for that. After I'd left the hospital, my unconscious mind was as unhappy with what had happened as my conscious one. Year after year, without my being aware, it had pondered those experiences, looking for meaning and drawing lessons. When I began to write, what came out was almost fully formed. This book had been written deep inside me.

Think back, and you'll see what I mean. What you've been reading is a snapshot of how almost every imaginable teen girl reacts to the embarrassments of hospitalization. I didn't plan that and, had I tried to write this book just after I left the hospital, I don't think I could have done it. Recall the girls we've met.

The Girls In This Story

Frightened little Min was so terrified that something might show, that to this day I don't know how I could have comforted her. She represents all those girls who enter a hospital absolutely terrified at their loss of control and the embarrassment that accompanies that. More than the others, this book is written for them. But for the kindness of individual staff acting on their own, nothing is done to protect such girls. Many hospitals have a VIP status that can be assigned to someone who is to get special treatment, perhaps because he has given the hospital buckets of money. I doubt any hospital has a VSG—Very Sensitive Girl status. They should.

Maria stands for innocence and trust. That's why I believe she was unharmed by what her nurse and I did that night. She trusted us and that was enough. But we should remember that same innocence could set her up to be the victim of someone perverted enough to know how to twist the rules. Again, it's difficult to see much hospitals are doing to prevent that, especially given that pernicious 'staff are not male or female' rule.

Yes, everything went well with Christy, illustrating that my successes tended to come with my most difficult situations. But something about those nights still bothers me. Her last days were safe because there was little risk that a guy working nights caring for little children with leukemia would be a creep. But suppose, I asked myself back then, she'd come from a poor family and was dying in the back ward of a badly run city hospital. Her last nights might have been a torment. That should never be.

Next are those amazing Post-Op Girls. I did my best to bring out the humor in their situation despite the frustrations they caused me. Taught too-casual practices by their first set of nurses, they embarrassed me more than they did themselves. But they do illustrate that hospitals need to rethink their obsession with single, overly efficient, unisex procedures. Hospitals need to make practical adjustments for men caring for teen girls and perhaps women caring for teen boys. I suspect the result wouldn't take that much more time.

Nor should we forget those most clever Sensible Girls—the ones I imagine are most like you, especially after you've read this book. They represent patients who're smart enough to work around a hospital's deficiencies, managing to stay comfortable during their stay while avoiding most embarrassments. In fact, they taught me more about teen-girl care than the hospital did. Hospitals should learn from them.

Then there were Heidi and the Twins, experienced patients who laid down firm guy-with-girl rules. They let me know where I stood and I appreciated that. Some hospital staff fear that, if rules like those of these girls became more common, patient care would descend into chaos. I doubt that. We easily adapted to those girls and could have adjusted to more like them. Learning how to be comfortable in a hospital shouldn't take numerous visits over a span of years. It should be the right of every patient, however new and helpless.

Next were two girls who left me with the greatest sense of pain, Pala and Tina. What almost happened to Pala and what did happen to Tina should not be happening in hospitals—not ever. The more vulnerable a patient is, due to a life-threatening illness, the more she should be protected from violation.

Young and defenseless, Pala was so overwhelmed by her recent diagnosis that she was dependent on me to do the right thing. But what's right should not hinge on an accidental pairing between someone experienced in the horrors of leukemia and someone facing those horrors for the first time. Kindness about embarrassment should be such a core value in hospitals, that everyone thinks about it and no one gets berated for acting on. There are more important things than bed sheets and efficiency, particularly for someone facing the serious possibility of dying.

Broken-spirited Tina illustrates that a hospital can fail almost criminally. Are girls around puberty particularly sensitive to violations of their modesty? I don't know, and I found no research on the topic. But I do know that a hospital's efforts to get patients to comply with intrusive procedures should never resemble the nasty techniques used by to force young teens into prostitution. The issue isn't that treatments for leukemia include such violations as a part of their written treatment protocols. That isn't true. It's that little or no effort has been made to ensure that this unconscious abuse of the vulnerable doesn't happen. We should be gentler with teens facing terrible illnesses and not add to their already heavy burdens.

It's also true that at times I was innocent of even a blunder. Ginny's embarrassment at being topless came from a nurse's misbehavior and not my own. I turned away as quickly as I could. Yet she was embarrassed none the less by me. Like Miss Buns and the Wet Hens, not everything was under my control. But much is under the control of hospital administrators and nursing instructors. Female staff can be taught not to be so cavalier with their female patients and male staff with male patients. A hospital is a terrible place to be when you're sick partly because of this woeful lack of privacy. It can be better.

Oddly, the two situations that came out best, caring for Christy as she lay dying and getting Jennie into a warm bath, were the ones that meant the most exposure for the girls involved. I can only attribute those successes to the fact that, even though words weren't spoken, both those girls and I knew we needed to work together. We established trust and that made all the difference. Trust even managed to trump the usual lack of communication. Hospitals need to encourage more of both.

That said, I fear that, in all too many situations, problems arose and issues were left unresolved because all talk about modesty, embarrassment, and even feelings of violation were taboo. Nursing staff, including me, seemed afraid to bring them up and expose their supposed lack of professionalism and insufficient desensitization. On their part, administrators seemed to fear that any lessening of the 'staff are neither male nor female' rule would complicate their work and lower efficiency. I doubt that's true.

Perhaps worst of all, those who should have been overseeing this, the hospital's senior physicians and nursing administrators, seemed to unable to see any patient issue that didn't fit with their mechanistic/scientific, diagnosis/treatment, drugs/surgery, staff/tasks, or budget/analysis modes of thinking.

Carina illustrates that in the grimmest of terms. She was much more than an nasty infection to be cured by antibiotics. Her issues ran far deeper and needed to be dealt with by involving her family, particularly her mother. Medicine also needs to learn to think about teen sexuality with honesty and sanity rather than just drugs and surgeries.

In short, I believe much of what goes on in hospitals needs to change. Feelings such as embarrassment do matter. Dealing with them should be as much a part of good medical care as pain management. No teen girl—including especially you—should be expected to set well-established feelings about embarrassment and modesty aside simply because

Hospital Gowns and Other Embarrassments

she's sick, much less because she has a potentially fatal illness. Kindness and gentleness are as important as survival rates.

In closing, I'd like to thank you for kindly staying with me through this book. I really do hope it helps make your hospital stay more pleasant and free of embarrassment. Remember, you're at the very heart of my hope for seeing change brought to hospitals. What you do not only changes how you're treated, it influences how other girls will be treated.

One final note. I'm an independent writer who has published this book myself. I need people like you to make it widely read. If you find it helpful, review it at online stores, recommend it to your friends, suggest that public and school libraries get copies, and perhaps persuade the gift store at your hospital to carry it. By doing that, you help other girls much like you.

CPSIA information can be obtained at www.ICGtesting.com
Printed in the USA
LVOW051314290413

331370LV00005B/352/P